YOGA ANATOMY

Leslie Kaminoff

Asana Analysis by
Amy Matthews

Illustrated by
Sharon Ellis

Human Kinetics

Library of Congress Cataloging-in-Publication Data

Kaminoff, Leslie.
  Yoga anatomy / Leslie Kaminoff ; illustrated by Sharon Ellis.
      p. cm.
  Includes indexes.
  ISBN-13: 978-0-7360-6278-7 (soft cover)
  ISBN-10: 0-7360-6278-5 (soft cover)
  1. Hatha yoga. 2. Human anatomy. I. Title.
  RA781.7.K356 2007
  613.7'046--dc22

                                                                2007010050

ISBN-10: 0-7360-6278-5
ISBN-13: 978-0-7360-6278-7

Acquisitions Editor: Martin Barnard
Developmental Editor: Leigh Keylock
Assistant Editor: Christine Horger
Copyeditor: Patsy Fortney
Proofreader: Kathy Bennett
Graphic Designer: Fred Starbird
Graphic Artist: Tara Welsch
Original Cover Designer: Lydia Mann
Cover Revisions: Keith Blomberg
Art Manager: Kelly Hendren
Project Photographer: Lydia Mann
Illustrator (cover and interior): Sharon Ellis. All illustrations © Sharon Ellis 2007.
Printer: United Graphics

Human Kinetics books are available at special discounts for bulk purchase. Special editions or book excerpts can also be created to specification. For details, contact the Special Sales Manager at Human Kinetics.

Printed in the United States of America   10   9   8

The paper in this book is certified under a sustainable forestry program.

Human Kinetics
Web site: www.HumanKinetics.com

United States: Human Kinetics
P.O. Box 5076
Champaign, IL 61825-5076
800-747-4457
e-mail: humank@hkusa.com

Canada: Human Kinetics
475 Devonshire Road, Unit 100
Windsor, ON N8Y 2L5
800-465-7301 (in Canada only)
e-mail: info@hkcanada.com

Europe: Human Kinetics
107 Bradford Road
Stanningley
Leeds LS28 6AT, United Kingdom
+44 (0)113 255 5665
e-mail: hk@hkeurope.com

Australia: Human Kinetics
57A Price Avenue
Lower Mitcham, South Australia 5062
08 8372 0999
e-mail: info@hkaustralia.com

New Zealand: Human Kinetics
Division of Sports Distributors NZ Ltd.
P.O. Box 300 226 Albany
North Shore City, Auckland
0064 9 448 1207
e-mail: info@humankinetics.co.nz

To my teacher, T.K.V. Desikachar, I offer this book in gratitude for his unwavering insistence that I find my own truth. My greatest hope is that this work can justify his confidence in me.

And, to my philosophy teacher, Ron Pisaturo—the lessons will never end.

—*Leslie Kaminoff*

In gratitude to all the students and teachers who have gone before . . . especially Philip, my student, teacher, and friend.

—*Amy Matthews*

CONTENTS

ACKNOWLEDGMENTS

First and foremost, I wish to express my gratitude to my family—my wife Uma, and my sons Sasha, Jai, and Shaun. Their patience, understanding, and love have carried me through the three-year process of conceiving, writing, and editing this book. They have sacrificed many hours that they would otherwise have spent with me, and that's what made this work possible. I am thankful beyond measure for their support. I wish also to thank my father and mother for supporting their son's unconventional interests and career for the past four decades. Allowing a child to find his own path in life is perhaps the greatest gift that a parent can give.

This has been a truly collaborative project which would never have happened without the invaluable, ongoing support of an incredibly talented and dedicated team. Lydia Mann, whose most accurate title would be "Project and Author Wrangler" is a gifted designer, artist, and friend who guided me through every phase of this project: organizing, clarifying, and editing the structure of the book; shooting the majority of the photographs (including the author photos); designing the cover; introducing me to BackPack, a collaborative Web-based service from 37 Signals, which served as the repository of the images, text, and information that were assembled into the finished book. Without Lydia's help and skill, this book would still be lingering somewhere in the space between my head and my hard drive.

My colleague and collaborator Amy Matthews was responsible for the detailed and innovative asana analysis that forms the backbone of the book. Working with Amy continues to be one of the richest and most rewarding professional relationships I've ever had.

Sharon Ellis has proven to be a skilled, perceptive, and flexible medical illustrator. When I first recruited her into this project after admiring her work online, she had no familiarity with yoga, but before long, she was slinging the Sanskrit terms and feeling her way through the postures like a seasoned yoga adept.

This project would never have existed had it not been originally conceived by the team at Human Kinetics. Martin Barnard's research led to me being offered the project in the first place. Leigh Keylock and Jason Muzinic's editorial guidance and encouragement kept the project on track. I can't thank them enough for their support and patience, but mostly for their patience.

A very special thank you goes to my literary agent and good friend, Bob Tabian, who has been a steady, reliable voice of reason and experience. He's the first person who saw me as an author, and never lost his faith that I could actually be one.

For education, inspiration, and coaching along the way, I thank Swami Vishnu Devananda, Lynda Huey, Leroy Perry Jr., Jack Scott, Larry Payne, Craig Nelson, Gary Kraftsow, Yan Dhyansky, Steve Schram, William LeSassier, David Gorman, Bonnie Bainbridge Cohen, Len Easter, Gil Hedley, and Tom Myers. I also thank all my students and clients past and present for being my most consistent and challenging teachers.

A big thank you goes out to all the models who posed for our images: Amy Matthews, Alana Kornfeld, Janet Aschkenasy, Mariko Hirakawa (our cover model), Steve Rooney (who also donated the studio at International Center of Photography for a major shoot), Eden Kellner, Elizabeth Luckett, Derek Newman, Carl Horowitz, J. Brown, Jyothi Larson, Nadiya Nottingham, Richard Freeman, Arjuna, Eddie Stern, Shaun Kaminoff, and Uma McNeill. Thanks also go to the Krishnamacharya Yoga Mandiram for permission to use the iconic photographs of Sri T. Krishnamacharya as reference for the Mahamudra and Mulabandhasana drawings.

Invaluable support for this project was also provided by Jen Harris, Edya Kalev, Leandro Villaro, Rudi Bach, Jenna O'Brien, and all the teachers, staff, students, and supporters of The Breathing Project.

—*Leslie Kaminoff*

Thanks to Leslie for inviting me to be a part of it all . . . little did I know what that "cool idea" would become! Many thanks to all of the teachers who encouraged my curiosity and passion for understanding things: especially Alison West, for cultivating a spirit of exploration and inquiry in her yoga classes; Mark Whitwell, for constantly reminding me of what I already know about why I am a teacher; Irene Dowd, for her enthusiasm and precision; and Bonnie Bainbridge Cohen, who models the passion and compassion for herself and her students that lets her be such a gift as a teacher.

And I am hugely grateful to all the people and circles that have sustained me in the process of working on this book: my dearest friends Michelle and Aynsley; the summer BMC circle, especially our kitchen table circle, Wendy, Elizabeth, and Tarina; Kidney, and all the people I told to "stop asking!"; my family; and my beloved Karen, without whose love and support I would have been much more cranky.

—*Amy Matthews*

INTRODUCTION

This book is by no means an exhaustive, complete study of human anatomy or the vast science of yoga. No single book possibly could be. Both fields contain a potentially infinite number of details, both macro- and microscopic—all of which are endlessly fascinating and potentially useful in certain contexts. My intention is to present what I consider to be the key details of anatomy that are of the most value and use to people who are involved in yoga, whether as students or teachers.

To accomplish this, a particular context, or view, is necessary. This view will help sort out the important details from the vast sea of information available. Furthermore, such a view will help to assemble these details into an integrated view of our existence as "indivisible entities of matter and consciousness."[1]

The view of yoga used in this book is based on the structure and function of the human body. Because yoga practice emphasizes the relationship of the breath and the spine, I will pay particular attention to those systems. By viewing all the other body structures in light of their relationship to the breath and spine, yoga becomes the integrating principle for the study of anatomy. Additionally, for yoga practitioners, anatomical awareness is a powerful tool for keeping our bodies safe and our minds grounded in reality.

The reason for this mutually illuminating relationship between yoga and anatomy is simple: The deepest principles of yoga are based on a subtle and profound appreciation of how the human system is constructed. The subject of the study of yoga is the Self, and the Self is dwelling in a physical body.

The ancient yogis held the view that we actually possess three bodies: physical, astral, and causal. From this perspective, yoga anatomy is the study of the subtle currents of energy that move through the layers, or "sheaths," of those three bodies. The purpose of this work is to neither support nor refute this view. I wish only to offer the perspective that if you are reading this book, you possess a mind and a body that is currently inhaling and exhaling in a gravitational field. Therefore, you can benefit immensely from a process that enables you to think more clearly, breathe more effortlessly, and move more efficiently. This, in fact, will be our basic definition of yoga practice: the integration of mind, breath, and body.

This definition is the starting point of this book, just as our first experience of breath and gravity was the starting point of our lives on this planet.

The context that yoga provides for the study of anatomy is rooted in the exploration of how the life force expresses itself through the movements of the body, breath, and mind. The ancient and exquisite metaphorical language of yoga has arisen from the very real anatomical experimentations of millions of seekers over thousands of years. All these seekers shared a common laboratory—the human body. It is the intention of this book to provide a guided tour of this "lab" with some clear instructions for how the equipment works and which basic procedures can yield useful insights. Rather than being a how-to manual for the practice of a particular system of yoga, I hope to offer a solid grounding in the principles that underlie the physical practice of all systems of yoga.

---

[1] I'm inspired here by a famous quote from philosopher and novelist Ayn Rand: "You are an indivisible entity of matter and consciousness. Renounce your consciousness and you become a brute. Renounce your body and you become a fake. Renounce the material world and you surrender it to evil."

A key element that distinguishes yoga practice from gymnastics or calisthenics is the intentional integration of breath, posture, and movement. The essential yogic concepts that refer to these elements are beautifully expressed by a handful of coupled Sanskrit terms:

prana/apana
sthira/sukha
brahmana/langhana
sukha/dukha

To understand these terms, we must understand how they were derived in the first place: by looking at the most fundamental functional units of life. We will define them as we go along.

To grasp the core principles of both yoga and anatomy, we will need to reach back to the evolutionary and intrauterine origins of our lives. Whether we look at the simplest single-celled organisms or our own beginnings as newly conceived beings, we will find the basis for the key yogic metaphors that relate to all life and that illuminate the structure and function of our thinking, breathing, moving human bodies.

T he most basic unit of life, the cell, can teach you an enormous amount about yoga. In fact, the most essential yogic concepts can be derived from observing the cell's form and function. This chapter explores breath anatomy from a yogic perspective, using the cell as a starting point.

Yoga Lessons From a Cell

Cells are the smallest building blocks of life, from single-celled plants to multitrillion-celled animals. The human body, which is made up of roughly 100 trillion cells, begins as a single, newly fertilized cell.

A cell consists of three parts: the cell membrane, the nucleus, and the cytoplasm. The membrane separates the cell's external environment, which contains nutrients that the cell requires, from its internal environment, which consists of the cytoplasm and the nucleus. Nutrients have to get through the membrane, and once inside, the cell metabolizes these nutrients and turns them into the energy that fuels its life functions. As a result of this metabolic activity, waste gets generated that must somehow get back out through the membrane. Any impairment in the membrane's ability to let nutrients in or waste out will result in the death of the cell via starvation or toxicity. This observation that living things take in nutrients provides a good basis for understanding the term *prana*, which refers to what nourishes a living thing. *Prana* refers not only to what is brought in as nourishment but also to the *action* that brings it in.[1]

Of course, there has to be a complementary force. The yogic concept that complements prana is *apana*, which refers to what is eliminated by a living thing as well as the action of elimination.[2] These two fundamental yogic terms—prana and apana—describe the essential activities of life.

Successful function, of course, expresses itself in a particular form. Certain conditions have to exist in a cell for nutrition (prana) to enter and waste (apana) to exit. The membrane's structure has to allow things to pass in and out of it—it has to be permeable (see figure 1.1). It can't be so permeable, however, that the cell wall loses its integrity; otherwise, the cell will either explode from the pressures within or implode from the pressures outside.

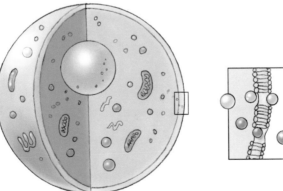

Figure 1.1　The cell's membrane must balance containment (stability) with permeability.

---

[1] The Sanskrit word *prana* is derived from *pra*, a prepositional prefix meaning "before," and *an*, a verb meaning "to breathe," "to blow," and "to live." Here, *prana* is not being capitalized, because it refers to the functional life processes of a single entity. The capitalized *Prana* is a more universal term that is used to designate the manifestation of all creative life force.

[2] The Sanskrit word *apana* is derived from *apa*, which means "away," "off," and "down," and *an*, which means "to blow," "to breathe," and "to live."

In the cell (and all living things, for that matter), the principle that balances permeability is stability. The yogic terms that reflect these polarities are *sthira*[3] and *sukha*.[4] All successful living things must balance containment and permeability, rigidity and plasticity, persistence and adaptability, space and boundaries.[5]

You have seen that observing the cell, the most basic unit of life, illuminates the most basic concepts in yoga: prana/apana and sthira/sukha. Next is an examination of the structure and function of the breath using these concepts as a guide.

Prana and Apana

The body's pathways for nutrients and waste are not as simple as those of a cell, but they are not so complex that you can't grasp the concepts as easily.

Figure 1.2 shows a simplified version of the nutritional and waste pathways. It shows how the human system is open at the top and at the bottom. You take in prana, nourishment, in solid and liquid form at the top of the system: It enters the alimentary canal, goes through the digestive process, and after a lot of twists and turns, the resulting waste moves down and out. It has to go down to get out because the exit is at the bottom. So, the force of apana, when it's acting on solid and liquid waste, has to move down to get out.

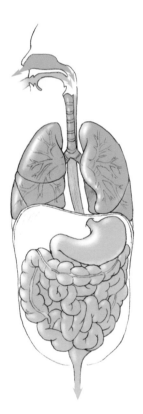

You also take in prana in gaseous form: The breath, like solid and liquid nutrition, enters at the top. But the inhaled air remains above the diaphragm in the lungs (see figure 1.3), where it exchanges gases with the capillaries at the alveoli. The waste gases in the lungs need to get out—but they need to get back out the same way they came in. This is why it is said that apana must be able to operate freely both upward and downward, depending on what type of waste it's acting on. That is also why any inability to reverse apana's downward push will result in an incomplete exhalation.

The ability to reverse apana's downward action is a very basic and useful skill that can be acquired through yoga training, but it is not something that most people are able to do right away. Pushing downward is the way that most people are accustomed to operating their apana because whenever there's anything within the body that needs to be disposed, humans tend to squeeze in and push down. That is why most beginning yoga students, when asked to exhale completely, will squeeze in and push down their breathing muscles as if they're urinating or defecating.

Figure 1.2   Solid and liquid nutrition (blue) enter at the top of the system and exit as waste at the bottom. Gaseous nutrition and waste (red) enter and exit at the top.

---

[3] The Sanskrit word *sthira* means "firm," "hard," "solid," "compact," "strong," "unfluctuating," "durable," "lasting," and "permanent." English words such as *stay*, *stand*, *stable*, and *steady* are likely derived from the Indo-European root that gave rise to the Sanskrit term.

[4] The Sanskrit word *sukha* originally meant "having a good axle hole," implying a space at the center that allows function; it also means "easy," "pleasant," "agreeable," "gentle," and "mild."

[5] Successful man-made structures also exhibit a balance of sthira and sukha; for example, a colander's holes that are large enough to let out liquid, but small enough to prevent pasta from falling through, or a suspension bridge that's flexible enough to survive wind and earthquake, but stable enough to support its load-bearing surfaces.

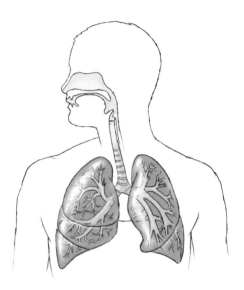

Figure 1.3   The pathway that air takes into and out of the body.

Sukha and Dukha

The pathways must be clear of obstructing forces in order for prana and apana to have a healthy relationship. In yogic language, this region must be in a state of *sukha*, which literally translates as "good space." "Bad space" is referred to as *dukha*, which is commonly translated as "suffering."[6]

This model points to the fundamental methodology of all classical yoga practice, which attends to the blockages, or obstructions, in the system to improve function. The basic idea is that when you make more "good space," your pranic forces will flow freely and restore normal function. This is in contrast to any model that views the body as missing something essential, which has to be added from the outside. This is why it has been said that yoga therapy is 90 percent about waste removal.

Another practical way of applying this insight to the field of breath training is the observation: If you take care of the exhalation, the inhalation takes care of itself.

Breathing, Gravity, and Yoga

Keeping in the spirit of starting from the beginning, let's look at some of the things that happen at the very start of life.

In utero, oxygen is delivered through the umbilical cord. The mother does the breathing. There is no air and very little blood in the lungs when in utero because the lungs are nonfunctional and mostly collapsed. The circulatory system is largely reversed, with oxygen-rich blood flowing through the veins and oxygen-depleted blood flowing through the arteries. Humans even have blood flowing through vessels that won't exist after birth, because they will seal off and become ligaments.

Being born means being severed from the umbilical cord—the lifeline that sustained you for nine months. Suddenly, and for the first time, you need to engage in actions that will ensure continued survival. The very first of these actions declares your physical and physiological independence. *It is the first breath*, and it is the most important and forceful inhalation you will ever take in your life.

That first inhalation was the most important one because the initial inflation of the lungs causes essential changes to the entire circulatory system, which had previously been geared toward receiving oxygenated blood from the mother. The first breath causes blood to surge into the lungs, the right and left sides of the heart to separate into two pumps, and the specialized vessels of fetal circulation to shut down and seal off.

That first inhalation is the most forceful one you will ever take because it needs to overcome the initial surface tension of your previously collapsed and amniotic-fluid-filled lung

---

[6] The Sanskrit word *sukha* is derived from *su* (meaning "good") and *kha* (meaning "space"). In this context (paired with dukha), it refers to a state of well-being, free of obstacles. Like the "good axle hole," a person needs to have "good space" at his or her center. The Sanskrit word *dukha* is derived from *dus* (meaning "bad") and *kha* (meaning "space"). It is generally translated as "suffering"; also, "uneasy," "uncomfortable," "unpleasant," and "difficult."

tissue. The force required (called negative inspiratory force) is three to four times greater than that of a normal inhalation.

Another first-time experience that occurs at the moment of birth is the weight of the body in space. Inside the womb, you're in a weightless, fluid-filled environment. Then, suddenly, your entire universe expands because you're out—you're free. Now, your body can move freely in space, your limbs and head can move freely in relation to your body, and you must be supported in gravity. Because adults are perfectly willing to swaddle babies and move them from place to place, stability and mobility may not seem to be much of an issue so early in life, but they are. The fact is, right away you have to start *doing* something—you have to find nourishment, which involves the complex action of simultaneously breathing, sucking, and swallowing. All of the muscles involved in this intricate act of survival also create your first postural skill—supporting the weight of the head. This necessarily involves the coordinated action of many muscles, and—as with all postural skills—a balancing act between mobilization and stabilization. Postural development continues from the head downward, until you begin walking (after about a year), culminating with the completion of your lumbar curve (at about 10 years of age).

To summarize, the moment you're born, you're confronted by two forces that were not present in utero: breath and gravity. To thrive, you need to reconcile those forces for as long as you draw breath on this planet. The practice of yoga can be seen as a way of consciously exploring the relationship between breath and posture, so it's clear that yoga can help you to deal with this fundamental challenge.

To use the language of yoga, life on this planet requires an integrated relationship between breath (prana/apana) and posture (sthira/sukha). When things go wrong with one, by definition they go wrong with the other.

The prana/apana concept is explored with a focus on the breathing mechanism. Chapter 2 covers the sthira/sukha concept by focusing on the spine. The rest of the book examines how the breath and spine come together in the practice of yoga postures.

Breathing Defined

Breathing is the process of taking air into and expelling it from the lungs. This is a good place to start, but let's define the "process" being referred to. Breathing—the passage of air into and out of the lungs—is movement, one of the fundamental activities of living things. Specifically, breathing involves movement in two cavities.

Movement in Two Cavities

The simplified illustration of the human body in figure 1.4 shows that the torso consists of two cavities, the thoracic and the abdominal. These cavities share some properties, and they have important distinctions as well. Both contain vital organs: The thoracic contains the heart and lungs, and the abdominal contains the stomach, liver, gall bladder, spleen, pancreas, small and large intestines, kidneys, and bladder, among others. Both cavities are bounded posteriorly by the spine. Both open at one end to the external environment—the thoracic at the top, and the abdominal at the bottom. Both share an important structure, the diaphragm (it forms the roof of the abdominal cavity and the floor of the thoracic cavity).

Another important shared property of the two cavities is that they are mobile—they change shape. It is this shape-changing ability that is most relevant to breathing, because without this movement, the body cannot breathe at all. Although both the abdominal and thoracic cavities change shape, there is an important structural difference in how they do so.

The abdominal cavity changes shape like a flexible, fluid-filled structure such as a water balloon. When you squeeze one end of a water balloon, the other end bulges. That is

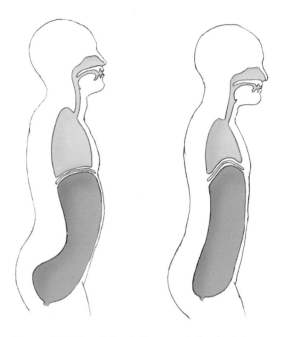

Figure 1.4 Breathing is thoracoabdominal shape change. Inhalation on left, exhalation on right.

because water is noncompressible. Your hand's action only moves the fixed volume of water from one end of the flexible container to the other. The same principle applies when the abdominal cavity is compressed by the movements of breathing; a squeeze in one region produces a bulge in another. That is because in the context of breathing, the abdominal cavity changes shape, but not volume.

In the context of life processes other than breathing, the abdominal cavity *does* change volume. If you drink a gallon of liquid or eat a big meal, the overall volume of the abdominal cavity will increase as a result of expanded abdominal organs (stomach, intestines, bladder). Any increase of volume in the abdominal cavity will produce a corresponding decrease in the volume of the thoracic cavity. That is why it's harder to breathe after a big meal, before a big bowel movement, or when pregnant.

In contrast to the abdominal cavity, the thoracic cavity changes both shape and volume; it behaves as a flexible gas-filled container, similar to an accordion bellows. When you squeeze an accordion, you create a reduction in the volume of the bellows and air is forced out. When you pull the bellows open, its volume increases and the air is pulled in. This is because the accordion is compressible and expandable. The same is true of the thoracic cavity, which, unlike the abdominal cavity and its contents, can change its shape *and* volume.

Volume and Pressure

Volume and pressure are inversely related: When volume increases, pressure decreases, and when volume decreases, pressure increases. Because air always flows toward areas of lower pressure, increasing the volume inside the thoracic cavity (think of an accordion) will decrease pressure and cause air to flow into it. This is an inhalation.

It is interesting to note that in spite of how it feels when you inhale, you are not *pulling* air into the body. On the contrary, air is pushed into the body by atmospheric pressure that always surrounds you. The actual force that gets air into the lungs is outside of the body. The energy you expend in breathing produces a shape change that lowers the pressure in your chest cavity and permits the air to be pushed into the body by the weight of the planet's atmosphere.

Let's now imagine the thoracic and abdominal cavities as an accordion stacked on top of a water balloon. This illustration gives a sense of the relationship of the two cavities in breathing; movement in one will necessarily result in movement in the other. Recall that during an inhalation (the shape change permitting air to be pushed into the lungs by the planet's atmospheric pressure), the thoracic cavity expands its volume. This pushes downward on the abdominal cavity, which changes shape as a result of the pressure from above.

During relaxed, quiet breathing (such as while sleeping), an exhalation is a passive reversal of this process. The thoracic cavity and lung tissue—which have been stretched open during the inhalation—spring back to their initial volume, pushing the air out and returning the thoracic cavity to its previous shape. This is referred to as a *passive recoil*. Any reduction in the elasticity of these tissues will result in a reduction of the body's ability to exhale passively—leading to a host of respiratory problems.

In breathing patterns that involve active exhaling (such as blowing out candles, speaking, and singing, as well as various yoga exercises), the musculature surrounding the two cavities contracts in such a way that the abdominal cavity is pushed upward into the thoracic cavity, or the thoracic cavity is pushed downward into the abdominal cavity, or any combination of the two.

Three-Dimensional Shape Changes of Breathing

Because the lungs occupy a three-dimensional space in the thoracic cavity, when this space changes shape to cause air movement, it changes shape three-dimensionally. Specifically, an inhalation involves the chest cavity increasing its volume from top to bottom, from side to side, and from front to back, and an exhalation involves a reduction of volume in those three dimensions (see figure 1.5).

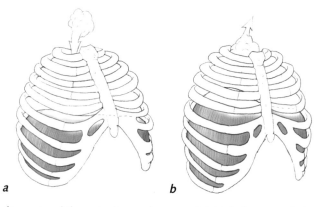

a   *b*

Figure 1.5   Three-dimensional thoracic shape changes of *(a)* inhalation and *(b)* exhalation.

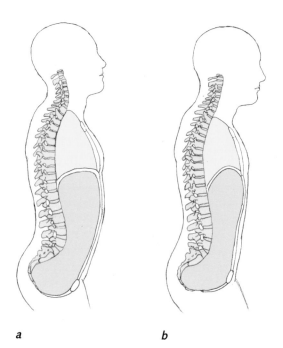

Because thoracic shape change is inextricably linked to abdominal shape change, you can also say that the abdominal cavity also changes shape (not volume) in three dimensions—it can be pushed or pulled from top to bottom, from side to side, or from front to back (see figure 1.6). In a living, breathing body, thoracic shape change cannot happen without abdominal shape change. That is why the condition of the abdominal region has such an influence on the quality of your breathing and why the quality of your breathing has a powerful effect on the health of your abdominal organs.

Figure 1.6   Changes in abdominal shape during breathing: *(a)* Inhalation = spinal extension; *(b)* exhalation = spinal flexion.

a   *b*

Expanded Definition of Breathing

Based on the information you have so far, here's an expanded definition of breathing:

Breathing, the process of taking air into and expelling it from the lungs, is caused by a three-dimensional changing of shape in the thoracic and abdominal cavities.

Defining breathing in this manner explains not only what it is but also how it is done. This has profound implications for yoga practice, because it can lead you to examine the supporting, shape-changing structure that occupies the back of the body's two primary cavities—the spine, which is covered in chapter 2.

To understand how a single muscle, the diaphragm, is capable of producing all this movement, you now examine it in detail.

Diaphragm's Role in Breathing

Just about every anatomy book describes the diaphragm as the principal muscle of breathing. Add the diaphragm to the shape-change definition of breathing to begin your exploration of this remarkable muscle:

The diaphragm is the principal muscle that causes three-dimensional shape change in the thoracic and abdominal cavities.

To understand how the diaphragm causes this shape change, you will examine its shape and location in the body, where it's attached, and what is attached to it, as well as its action and relationship to the other muscles of breathing.

Shape and Location

The diaphragm divides the torso into the thoracic and abdominal cavities. It is the floor of the thoracic cavity and the roof of the abdominal cavity. Its structure extends through a wide section of the body—the uppermost part reaches the space between the third and fourth ribs, and its lowest fibers attach to the front of the third lumbar vertebra; "nipple to navel" is one way to describe it.

The deeply domed shape of the diaphragm has evoked many images. Some of the most common are a mushroom, a jellyfish, a parachute, and a helmet. It's important to note that the shape of the diaphragm is created by the organs it encloses and supports. Deprived of its relationship with those organs, its dome would collapse, much like a stocking cap without a head in it. It is also evident that the diaphragm has an asymmetrical double-dome shape, with the right dome rising higher than the left. This is because the liver pushes up from below the right dome, and the heart pushes down from above the left dome.

Origin and Insertion

The lower edges of the diaphragm's circumference originate from three distinct regions: the bottom of the sternum, the base of the rib cage, and the front of the lower spine (see figure 1.7). These three regions form a continuous rim of attachment for the diaphragm. The only bony components of this rim are the back of the xiphoid process and the front surfaces of the first three lumbar vertebrae. The majority of the diaphragm (over 90 percent) originates on flexible tissue: the costal cartilage of ribs 6 through 10 and the arcuate ligaments, which bridge the span from the 10th rib's cartilage to the floating 11th and 12th ribs and from there to the spine.

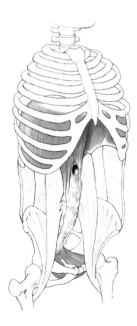

Figure 1.7　Origin and insertion of the diaphragm muscle.

All the muscular fibers of the diaphragm rise upward in the body from their origins. They eventually arrive at the flattened, horizontal top of the muscle, the central tendon, into which they insert. In essence, the diaphragm inserts into itself—its own central tendon, which is fibrous noncontractile tissue.

Organic Connections

The central tendon of the diaphragm is a point of anchorage for the connective tissue that surrounds the thoracic and abdominal organs. The names of these important structures are easily remembered as the three Ps.

- *Pleura*, which surround the lungs
- *Pericardium*, which surrounds the heart
- *Peritoneum*, which surrounds the abdominal organs

Thus, it should be clear that the shape-changing activity of these cavities has a profound effect on the movements of the organs they contain. The diaphragm is the primary source of these movements, and the relationship of its healthy functioning to the well-being of the organs is anatomically evident.

Actions

It is important to remember that the muscular fibers of the diaphragm are oriented primarily along the vertical (up–down) axis of the body, and this is the direction of the muscular action of the muscle. Recall that the horizontal central tendon is noncontractile and can move only in response to the action of the muscular fibers, which insert into it (see figure 1.8).

As in any other muscle, the contracting fibers of the diaphragm pull its insertion and origin (the central tendon and the base of the rib cage) toward each other. This muscle action is the fundamental cause of the three-dimensional thoracoabdominal shape changes of breathing.

To understand this fact more deeply, the question of whether origin moves toward insertion, or insertion moves toward origin, needs to be clarified. As with all muscles, the type of movement the diaphragm produces will depend on which end of the muscle is stable and which is mobile. To use an example of another muscle, the psoas muscle can create hip flexion either by moving the leg toward the front of the spine (as in standing on one leg and flexing the other hip) or by moving the front of the spine toward the leg (as in sit-ups with the legs braced). In both cases, the psoas muscle is doing the same thing—contracting. What differs is which end of the muscle is stable and which is mobile.

Just as you can think of the psoas as either a "leg mover" or a "trunk mover," you can think of the diaphragm as either a "belly bulger" or a "rib cage lifter" (see figure 1.9). The muscular action of the diaphragm is most often associated with a

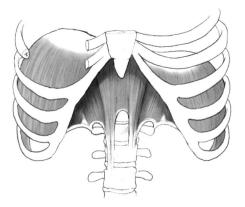

Figure 1.8 The muscle fibers of the diaphragm all run vertically from their origins to their insertion on the central tendon.

bulging[7] movement in the upper abdomen, which is commonly referred to as a "belly breath," but this is only the case if the diaphragm's origin (the base of the rib cage) is stable and its insertion (the central tendon) is mobile (see figure 1.10a).

If the central tendon is stabilized and the ribs are free to move, a diaphragmatic contraction will cause an expansion of the rib cage (see figure 1.10b). This is a "chest breath," which many people believe must be caused by the action of muscles other than the diaphragm. This mistaken idea can create a false dichotomy between diaphragmatic and "nondiaphragmatic" breathing. The unfortunate result of this error is that many people receiving breath training who exhibit chest movement (rather than belly movement) are told that they are not using the diaphragm, which is false. Except in cases of paralysis, the diaphragm is always used for breathing. The issue is whether it is being used efficiently.

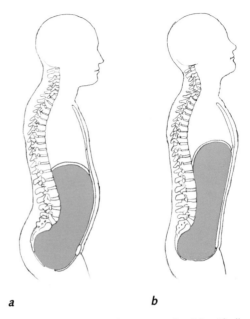

a   *b*

Figure 1.9 The diaphragm can be *(a)* a "belly bulger," during the belly inhalation, or *(b)* a "rib cage lifter," during the chest inhalation.

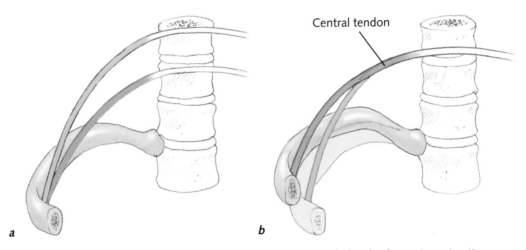

Central tendon

a   *b*

Figure 1.10 *(a)* With the rib stable and the abdominals relaxed, the diaphragm's contraction lowers the central tendon. *(b)* With the rib cage relaxed and the central tendon stabilized by abdominal action, the contracting diaphragm lifts the rib upward.

---

[7] Even though most teachers refer to this diaphragmatic action as an "expansion" of the abdomen, this is incorrect. In the context of breathing, the abdominal cavity does not change volume—only shape; therefore it is more accurate to refer to this movement as a "bulging" of the upper abdomen.

If it were possible to release all of the diaphragm's stabilizing muscles and allow its origin and insertion to freely move toward each other, both the chest and abdomen would move simultaneously. This rarely occurs because the need to stabilize the body's mass in gravity will cause many of the respiratory stabilizing muscles (which are also postural muscles) to remain active through all phases of breathing.

Engine of Three-Dimensional Shape Change

The diaphragm is the prime mover of the thoracic and abdominal cavities. The specific patterns that arise in yoga asana practice or breathing exercises, however, result from the action of muscles other than the diaphragm that can change the shape of the cavities. These are called *accessory muscles*. The analogy of a car and its engine is very useful in explaining this principle.

The engine is the prime mover of the car. All the movements associated with a car's operation (including the electrical) are generated in the engine. In the same manner, the three-dimensional, thoracoabdominal shape change of breathing is primarily generated by the diaphragm.

When you drive, the only direct control you exert over the function of the engine is the speed of its spinning. You push the gas pedal to make the engine spin faster, and you release the pedal to make it spin slower. Similarly, the only direct volitional control you have over the diaphragm is its timing.

You don't steer your car with its engine. To control the power of the engine and guide it in a particular direction, you need the mechanisms of the transmission, brakes, steering, and suspension. In the same way, you don't "steer" your breathing with the diaphragm. To control the power of the breath, and guide it into specific patterns, you need the assistance of the accessory muscles.

From the standpoint of this engine analogy, the whole notion of "diaphragmatic training" as a way to improve breath function is flawed. After all, you don't become a better driver by learning only how to work the gas pedal. Most of the skills you acquire in driver training have to do with getting the acceleration of the car to coordinate with steering, braking, and shifting gears. In a similar way, breath training is really "accessory muscle training." Once all the other musculature of the body is coordinated and integrated with the action of the diaphragm, breathing will be efficient and effective.

Additionally, the notion that that diaphragmatic action is limited to abdominal bulging (belly breathing) is as inaccurate as asserting that a car's engine is only capable of making it go forward—and that some other source of power must govern reverse movement. Just as this automotive error is linked to not understanding the relationship of the car's engine to its transmission, the breathing error results from not understanding the relationship of the diaphragm to the accessory muscles.

Moreover, equating belly movement with proper breathing and chest movement with improper breathing is just as silly as stating that a car is best served by only driving forward at all times. Without the ability to reverse its movements, a car would eventually end up someplace it couldn't get out of.

Accessory Muscles of Respiration

Although there is universal agreement that the diaphragm is the principal muscle of breathing, there are various, sometimes conflicting ways of categorizing the other muscles that participate in breathing. Using the definition of breathing as thoracoabdominal shape change, you can define *any* muscle other than the diaphragm that can cause a shape change in the cavities as accessory (see figures 1.11 and 1.12 for example). It's irrelevant whether the shape change leads to an increase or a decrease of thoracic volume (inhalation or exhalation), because both sets of muscles can be active during any phase of breathing. An example would be the analysis of a belly breath or a chest breath.

In the belly breath, the costal circumference (origin) of the diaphragm is stabilized by the muscles that pull the rib cage downward: the internal intercostals, the transversus thoracis, and others (see figures 1.13 to 1.16). These muscles are universally classified as "exhaling muscles," but here they actively participate in shaping an inhalation. In the chest breath, the central tendon (insertion) of the diaphragm is stabilized by the abdominal muscles, also regarded as "exhaling muscles," but in this case, they are clearly acting to produce a pattern of inhaling. It should be noted that in both of these cases, one region of accessory muscle has to be relaxed while the other is active. In the belly breath, the abdominal wall releases, and in the chest breath, the rib cage depressors have to let go.

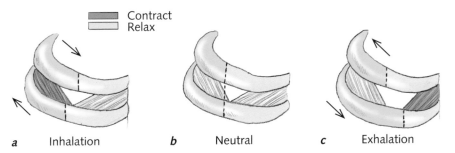

Contract
Relax

| *a* Inhalation | *b* Neutral | *c* Exhalation |

Figure 1.11   The intercostal muscles assist the sliding action of the ribs during respiration. During inhalation *(a)*, the external intercostals contract, and the internal intercostals relax. During exhalation *(c)*, the opposite occurs.

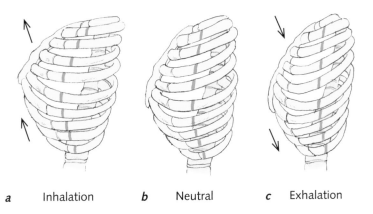

| *a* Inhalation | *b* Neutral | *c* Exhalation |

Figure 1.12   Contrary to appearances, the intercostal spaces remain constant during respiratory movements. Rather, the ribs slide in relation to each other—as indicated by the misaligning of the red line.

Abdominal and Thoracic Accessory Muscles

The abdominal cavity and its musculature can be imagined as a water balloon surrounded on all sides by elastic fibers running in all directions. The shortening and lengthening of these fibers in coordination with the contractions of the diaphragm produce the infinitely variable shape changes associated with respiration. As the tone of the diaphragm increases (inhalation), the tone of some abdominal muscles must decrease to allow the diaphragm to move. If you contract all your abdominal muscles at once and try to inhale, you'll notice that it's quite difficult because you've limited the ability of your abdomen to change shape.

The abdominal group doesn't affect breathing only by limiting or permitting shape change in the abdominal cavity. Because they also attach directly to the rib cage, the abdominal muscles directly affect its ability to expand.

The abdominal muscles that have the most direct effect on breathing are the ones that originate at the same place as the diaphragm, the transversus abdominis (see figure 1.13). This deepest layer of the abdominal wall arises from the costal cartilage at the base of the rib cage's inner surface. The fibers of the transversus are interdigitated (interwoven) at right angles with those of the diaphragm, whose fibers ascend vertically, whereas those of the transversus run horizontally (see figure 1.14). This makes the transversus abdominis the direct antagonist to the diaphragm's action of expanding the rib cage. The same layer of horizontal fibers extends upward into the posterior thoracic wall as the tranversus thoracis, a depressor of the sternum.

The other layers of the abdominal wall have similar counterparts in the thoracic cavity. The external obliques turn into the external intercostals, and the internal obliques turn into the internal intercostals (see figure 1.13). Of all these thoracoabdominal layers of muscle, only the external intercostals are capable of increasing thoracic volume. All the others produce a reduction of thoracic volume—either by depressing the rib cage or pushing upward on the central tendon of the diaphragm.

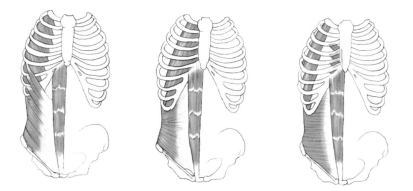

Figure 1.13 The continuity of the abdominal and intercostal layers shows how the external obliques turn into the external intercostals, internal obliques turn into the internal intercostals, and the transversus abdominis turns into the transversus thoracis and innermost intercostals.

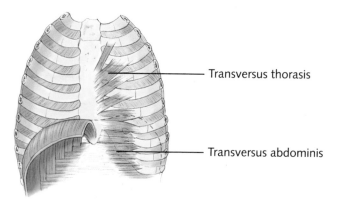

Transversus thorasis

Transversus abdominis

Figure 1.14 Posterior view of the chest wall, showing the interdigitated origins of the diaphragm and transversus abdominis forming perfect right angles with each other. This is clearly an agonist/antagonist, inhale/exhale muscle pairing that structurally underlies the yogic concepts of prana/apana.

Other Accessory Muscles

Chest, neck, and back muscles can expand the rib cage (see figures 1.15 and 1.16), but they are far more inefficient than the diaphragm and external intercostals at doing this. This inefficiency is the result of the fact that the location and attachment of these muscles do not provide enough leverage on the rib cage, and the usual role of these muscles is not respiration. They are primarily neck, shoulder girdle, and arm mobilizers—actions that require them to be stable proximally (toward the core of the body) and mobile distally (toward the periphery of the body). For these muscles to expand the rib cage, this relationship must be reversed—the distal insertions must be stabilized by yet more muscles so the proximal origins can be mobilized.

Considering the degree of muscular tension that accessory breathing entails, the net payoff in oxygenation makes it a poor energetic investment. That is why improved breathing is really a result of decreased tension in the accessory mechanism, which allows the diaphragm, with its shape-changing ability, to operate as efficiently as possible.

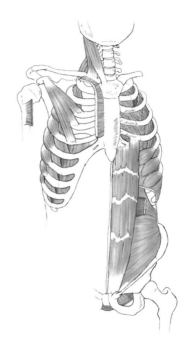

Figure 1.15 Some of the accessory muscles of respiration: Blue muscles act to reduce thoracic volume, while red muscles help to increase thoracic volume.

The Other Two Diaphragms

Along with the respiratory diaphragm, breathing involves the coordinated action of the pelvic and vocal diaphragms. Of particular interest to yoga practitioners is the action of mula bandha, which is a lifting action produced in the pelvic floor muscles (shown in figure 1.17, *a* and *b*) that also includes the lower fibers of the deep abdominal layers. Mula bandha is an action that moves apana upward and stabilizes the central tendon of the diaphragm. Inhaling while this bandha is active requires a release of the attachments of the upper abdominal wall, which permits the diaphragm to lift the base of the rib cage upward. This action is referred to as uddiyana bandha (*uddiya* means "flying upward").

It's important to note that the more superficial muscular fibers of the perineum need not be involved in mula bandha, because they contain the anal and urethral sphincters, which are associated with the downward movement of apana (elimination of solid and liquid waste), as shown in figure 1.18.

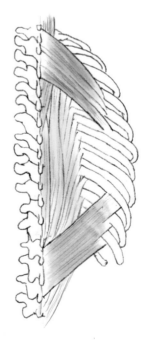

Figure 1.16 The serratus posterior muscles: superior (red) assist thoracic volume expansion, inferior (blue) assist thoracic volume reduction.

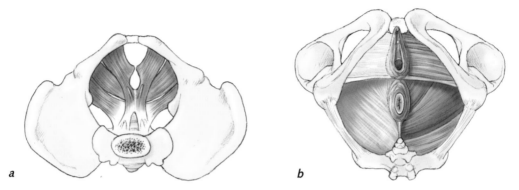

a   b

Figure 1.17   *(a)* The deepest muscles of the pelvic diaphragm, from above. *(b)* The pelvic floor from below, showing the orientation of superficial and deeper layers. The more superficial the layer, the more it runs from side to side (ischia to ischia); the deeper the layer, the more it runs front to back (pubic joint to coccyx).

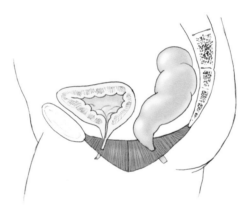

Figure 1.18   The action of the more superficial perineal fibers (figure 1.17*b*) are associated with the anal and urogenital sphincters and the downward movement of apana (i.e., the elimination of solid and liquid waste). The action of deeper fibers of the pelvic diaphragm (figure 1.17*a*) are associated with the upward movement of apana (i.e., the elimination of gaseous waste through exhalation).

Vocal Diaphragm

The gateway to the respiratory passages is the glottis, shown in figure 1.19, which is not a structure but a space between the vocal folds (cords). Yoga practitioners are accustomed to regulating this space in various ways, based on what they are doing with their breath, voice, and posture. When at rest, the muscles that control the vocal cords can be relaxed so that the glottis is being neither restricted nor enlarged (see figure 1.20*a*). This occurs in sleep and in the more restful, restorative practices in yoga.

When doing breathing exercises that involve deep, rapid movements of breath (such as kapalabhati or bhastrika), the muscles that pull the vocal folds apart contract to create a larger passage for the air movements (see figure 1.20*b*). When the exercises call for long, deep, slow breaths, the glottis can be partially closed, with only a small opening at the back of the cords (see figure 1.20*c*). This is the same action that creates whispered speech; in yoga it's known as *ujjayi*,[8] "the victorious breath."

---

[8] *U* denotes *udana*, which refers to the upward flowing prana in the throat region. *Jaya* means "victory."

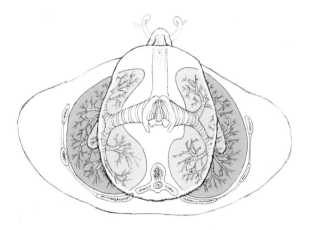

Figure 1.19   The pathway of air (in blue) into and out of the lungs.

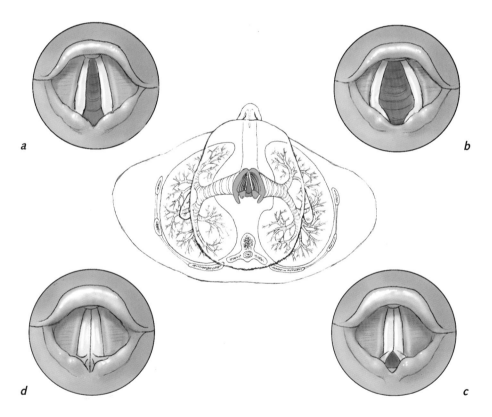

Figure 1.20   Position and location of vocal folds: *(a)* relaxed position, *(b)* maximal opening for forced respiration, *(c)* slightly opened for whispered speech (or *ujjayi*), *(d)* closed for speaking (phonation).

When making sound and during the chanting practices of yoga, the cords are pulled together into the phonation position (see figure 1.20*d*). The air pushing its way through them vibrates, creating sound. The pitch (and to some extent the length) of the sound is determined by how much tension is used to hold the cords together.

The Bandhas

All three diaphragms (pelvic, respiratory, and vocal) plus ujjayi come together in yoga movements that are coordinated with inhaling and exhaling. In addition to giving more length and texture to the breath, the "valve" of ujjayi creates a kind of back pressure throughout the abdominal and thoracic cavities that can protect the spine during the long, slow flexion and extension movements that occur in vinyasas such as the sun salutations. In yogic terms, these actions of the diaphragms (bandhas) create more sthira (stability) in the body, protecting it from injury by redistributing mechanical stress. An additional effect of moving the body through this resistance is the creation of heat in the system, which can be used in many beneficial ways. These practices are referred to as *brahmana*,[9] which implies heat, expansion, and the development of power and strength as well as the ability to withstand stress. Brahmana is also associated with inhaling, nourishment, prana, and the chest region.

When relaxing the body in the more supported, horizontal, restorative practices, remember to release the bandhas and glottal constrictions that are associated with vertical postural support. This relaxing side of yoga embodies the qualities of *langhana*,[10] which is associated with coolness, condensation, relaxation, and release as well as the development of sensitivity and inward focus. Langhana is also associated with exhaling, elimination, apana, and the abdominal region.

Because the ultimate goal of yoga breath training is to free up the system from habitual, dysfunctional restrictions, the first thing you need to do is free yourself from the idea that there's a single right way to breathe. As useful as the bandhas are when supporting your center of gravity and moving the spine through space, you need to release the forces of sthira in the system when pursuing the relaxation and release of sukha.

If yoga practice leads you to more integrated, balanced breathing, it's because it trains your body to freely respond to the demands that you place on it in the various positions and activities that make up your daily life.

---

[9] The Sanskrit root *brh* can mean "to grow great or strong," "increase," "to make big or fat or strong," and "expand."

[10] *Langhana* is a term that originates in Ayurveda, the ancient Indian system of medicine, and it refers to practices such as fasting that reduce, or eliminate, elements from the system.

The central nervous system, with its complex sensory and motor functions, allows for an enormous amount of flexibility in a vertebrate's survival activities. As these systems evolved over millions of years and became more crucial to the survival of our early ancestors, they required the corresponding development of a protective structure that allows for free movement but is stable enough to offer protection to these vital yet delicate tissues. That structure, the skeletal spine, is perhaps nature's most elegant and intricate solution to the dual demands of sthira and sukha.

The human spine is unique among all mammals in that it exhibits both primary and secondary curves. The primary curve of the spine comprises the kyphotic thoracic and sacral curves; the secondary, lordotic curves are present in the cervical and lumbar regions (see figure 2.1). Only a true biped requires both pairs of curves; tree-swinging and knuckle-walking primates have some cervical curve, but no lumbar lordosis, which is why they can't walk comfortably on two legs for long.

The primary (kyphotic) curve was the first front–back[1] spinal curve to emerge as aquatic creatures made the transition to land. As a human awaits its emergence from its watery origins in utero, the entire spine is in a primary curve (see figure 2.2). It changes shape for the first time when the head negotiates the hairpin curve of the birth canal and the neck experiences its secondary (lordotic) curve for the very first time[2] (see figure 2.3).

As your postural development proceeds from the head downward, the cervical curve continues to develop after you learn to hold up the weight of your head at about three to four months and fully forms at around nine months, when you learn to sit upright (see figure 2.4).

After crawling and creeping on the floor for months, you must acquire a lumbar curve to bring your weight over the feet. At 12 to 18 months, as you begin to walk, the lumbar spine straightens out from its primary, kyphotic curve. By 3 years of age, the lumbar spine starts to become concave forward (lordotic), although this won't be outwardly visible until 6 to 8 years of age. It is only after the age of 10 that the lumbar curve fully assumes its adult shape.

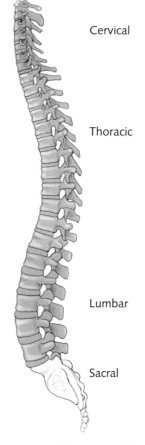

Cervical

Thoracic

Lumbar

Sacral

Figure 2.1 The curves of the spinal column.

---

[1] The lateral undulations that propel fish, snakes, and lizards through their environments cease to be useful for a creature that supports its belly off the ground on four limbs. The successful early quadrupeds would have been those that arched their bellies away from the earth so that their weight-bearing and movement forces were distributed into the limbs and away from the vulnerable center of the spine.

[2] This parallels the fact that the cervical spine was the site of the first development of a secondary curve as our quadrupedal ancestors found a survival benefit to lifting their heads and gazing from the ground immediately in front of them, out to the horizon.

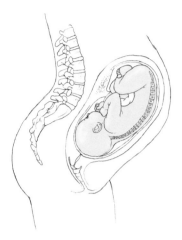

Figure 2.2   The entire spine exhibiting the primary curve in utero.

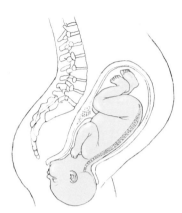

Figure 2.3   The first emergence of the secondary curve: negotiating the 90-degree turn from the cervix into the vaginal passage.

Birth   3 to 9 months   1 to 3 years   6 to 10 years

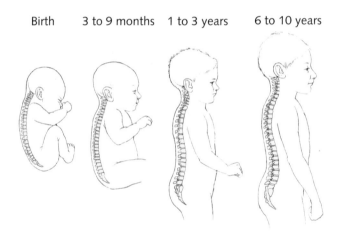

Figure 2.4   Development of primary and secondary curves.

The full glory of nature's ingenuity is apparent in the human spine—more so than in any other vertebrate structure. From an engineering perspective, it's clear that humans have the smallest base of support, the highest center of gravity, and the heaviest brain (proportional to total body weight[3]) of any other mammal. As the only true biped mammals on the planet, humans are also earth's least mechanically stable creatures. Fortunately, the disadvantage of having a bowling-ball-weighted cranium balancing on top of the whole system is offset by the advantage of having that big brain; it can figure out how to make the whole thing work efficiently—and that's where yoga can help.

The human form in general, and the spine in particular, exhibits an extraordinary resolution between the contradictory requirements of rigidity and plasticity. As you will see in the next section, the structural balancing of the forces of sthira and sukha in your living body relates to a principle called intrinsic equilibrium—a deep source of support that can be uncovered through yoga practice.

---

[3] The blue whale has the biggest brain on the planet, but it comprises only .01 percent of its total body weight. Humans top the list at 1.9 percent, with the rat a close second at 1.5 percent.

Intrinsic Equilibrium

If you were to remove all the muscles that attach to the spine, it still would not collapse. Why? Intrinsic equilibrium is the concept that explains not only why the spine is a self-supporting structure but also why any spinal movement produces potential energy that returns the spine to neutral. The same arrangement exists in the rib cage and pelvis, which, like the spine, are bound together under mechanical tension. This fact about the core structures of the axial skeleton reveals a deeper truth about how yoga practice appears to liberate potential energy from the body.

True to the principles of yoga and yoga therapy, the most profound changes occur when the forces obstructing that change are reduced. In the case of intrinsic equilibrium, a deep level of built-in support for the core of the body is involved. This built-in support does not depend on muscular effort because it is derived from the relationships between the non-contractile tissues of cartilage, ligament, and bone. Consequently, when this support asserts itself, it is always because some extraneous muscular effort has ceased to obstruct it.

It takes a lot of energy to fuel our constant, unconscious muscular exertions against gravity, and that is why the release of that effort is associated with a feeling of liberated energy. Thus, it is tempting to refer to intrinsic equilibrium as a source of energy because its discovery is always accompanied by a profound sensation of increased vitality in the body. In short, yoga can help you to release the stored potential energy of the axial skeleton by identifying and releasing the less efficient extraneous muscular effort that can obstruct the expression of those deeper forces.

Elements of Linkage Between the Vertebrae

The spinal column as a whole is ideally constructed to neutralize the combination of compressive and tensile forces to which it is constantly subjected by gravity and movement. The 24 vertebrae are bound to each other with intervening zones of cartilaginous discs, capsular joints, and spinal ligaments (shown schematically in blue in figure 2.5). This alternation of bony and soft tissue structures represents a distinction between passive and active elements; the vertebrae are the passive, stable elements (sthira), and the active, moving elements (sukha) are the intervertebral discs, facet (capsular) joints, and a network of ligaments that connect the arches of adjacent vertebrae (figure 2.6). The intrinsic equilibrium of the spinal column can be found in the integration of these passive and active elements.

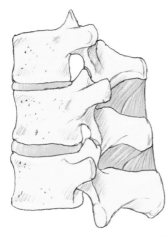

Figure 2.5 Alternating zones of hard and soft tissue in the spinal column.

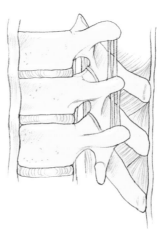

Figure 2.6 Ligaments of the spine.

To understand the overall architecture of the spine, it is useful to view it as two separate columns. In the schematic side view in figure 2.7, its front-to-back dimension can be roughly divided in half between a column of vertebral bodies and a column of arches.

Functionally, this arrangement very clearly evolved to contend with the dual requirements of stability and plasticity. The anterior column of vertebral bodies deals with weight-bearing, compressive forces, whereas the posterior column of arches deals with the tensile forces generated by movement. Within each column, in the dynamic relationship of bone to soft tissue, there is a balance of sthira and sukha. The vertebral bodies transmit compressive forces to the discs, which resist compression by pushing back. The column of arches transmits tension forces to all the attached ligaments (figure 2.8), which resist stretching by pulling back. In short, the structural elements of the spinal column are involved in an intricate dance that protects the central nervous system by neutralizing the forces of tension and compression.

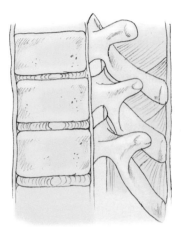

Figure 2.7   Viewed from the side, the spine divided into an anterior column of vertebral bodies and discs, and a posterior column of arches and processes.

Discs and Ligaments

If you look deeper, you can also see how sthira and sukha are revealed in the components of an intervertebral disc: The tough, fibrous layers of the annulus fibrosis tightly enclose the soft, spherical nucleus pulposus. In a healthy disc, the nucleus is completely contained all around by the annulus and the vertebra (see figure 2.9). The annulus fibrosis is itself contained front and back by the anterior and posterior longitudinal ligaments, with which it is closely bonded (see figure 2.8).

This tightly contained arrangement results in a strong tendency for the nucleus to always return to the center of the disc, no matter in which direction the body's movements propel it.

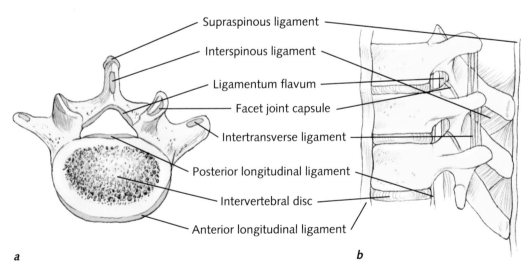

Supraspinous ligament
Interspinous ligament
Ligamentum flavum
Facet joint capsule
Intertransverse ligament
Posterior longitudinal ligament
Intervertebral disc
Anterior longitudinal ligament

a   *b*

Figure 2.8   *(a)* Superior view of spinal ligaments, and *(b)* lateral view of spinal ligaments.

Vertebral Structure

From the top of the cervical spine to the base of the lumbar spine, individual vertebrae are dramatically different in shape based on the functional demands of the varying regions of the spine (figure 2.10). There are, however, common elements to all vertebral structure, as illustrated by the schematic representation in figure 2.11.

Weight-bearing activities in general, as well as axial rotation (twisting movements), produce symmetrical (axial) compressive forces that flatten the nucleus into the annulus, which pushes back, resulting in a decompressive reaction (see figure 2.12). If the compressive force is high enough, rather than rupture, the nucleus will lose some of its moisture to the porous bone of the vertebral body. When the weight is taken

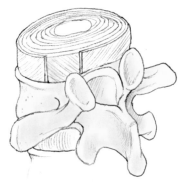

Figure 2.9 The nucleus pulposus is tightly bound by the annulus fibrosis, which contains concentric rings of oblique fibers that alternate their direction—similar to the internal and external abdominal obliques.

off the spine, the hydrophilic nucleus draws the water back in, and the disc returns to its original thickness. That is why humans are a bit taller right after getting out of bed.

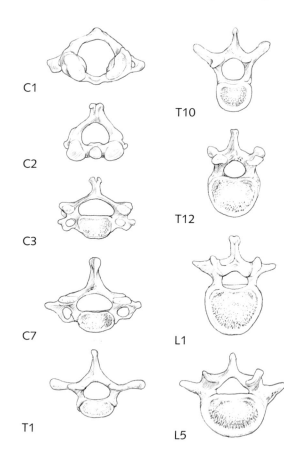

C1

C2

C3

C7

T1

T10

T12

L1

L5

Figure 2.10 The changing shape of the vertebrae.

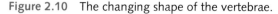

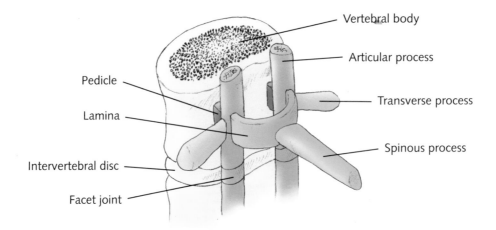

Vertebral body

Articular process

Pedicle

Transverse process

Lamina

Spinous process

Intervertebral disc

Facet joint

Figure 2.11 Common elements of a vertebra's structure.

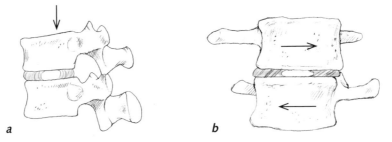

a

b

Figure 2.12 Weight-bearing forces *(a)* as well as twisting *(b)* produce symmetrical compression (flattening) of the nucleus, which, under pressure from the annulus, returns to its spherical shape, thus decompressing the vertebrae.

The movements of flexion, extension, and lateral flexion produce asymmetrical movements of the nucleus, but the result is the same: Wherever the vertebral bodies move toward each other, the nucleus is pushed in the opposite direction, where it meets the counterpush of the annulus, which causes the nucleus to push the vertebral bodies back to neutral (see figure 2.13).

Assisting in this counterpush are the long ligaments that run the entire length of the spine, front and back. The anterior longitudinal ligament runs all the way from the upper front of the sacrum to the front of the occiput, and it is fixed tightly to the front surface of each intervertebral disc. When it is stretched during backward bending, not only does

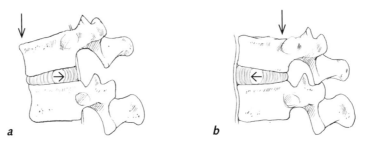

a

b

Figure 2.13 Flexion *(a)* and extension *(b)* movements produce asymmetrical movements of the nucleus, which, under pressure from the annulus, returns to a central position, thus helping the spine to return to neutral.

it tend to spring the body back to neutral, but the increased tension at its attachment to the disc also helps to propel the nucleus back to neutral. The opposite action occurs in the posterior longitudinal ligament when it is stretched in a forward bend. It runs from the back of the sacrum to the back of the occiput.

Every movement that produces disc compression in the anterior column necessarily results in tension to corresponding ligaments attached to the posterior column. The recoiling of these ligaments out of their stretched state adds to the other forces of intrinsic equilibrium, which combine to return the spine to neutral.

Note that all this activity occurs in tissues that behave independently of the circulatory, muscular, and voluntary nervous systems. In other words, their actions do not present an energy demand on these other systems.

Types of Spinal Movement

There are generally thought to be four possible movements of the spine: flexion, extension, axial rotation (twisting), and lateral flexion (side bending). These four movements occur more or less spontaneously in the course of life: as you bend over to tie your shoes (flexion), reach for something on a high shelf (extension), grab a bag in the car seat behind you (axial rotation), or reach your arm into the sleeve of an overcoat (lateral flexion). There are, of course, yoga postures that emphasize these movements as well.

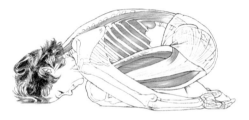

A more thorough look into the nature of the four ranges of motion of the spine shows that there is a fifth possibility called axial extension. This motion doesn't happen spontaneously in the normal course of daily movements. You have to learn how to make it happen intentionally because it is somewhat unnatural.

Figure 2.14 Child's pose replicates the primary curve of the unborn child.

Flexion and Extension, the Primary and Secondary Curves, and Inhalation and Exhalation

The most basic movement of the spine is the one that emphasizes its primary curve: flexion. As discussed previously, the primary curve is the kyphotic curve present primarily in the thoracic spine, but it is also obvious in the shape of the sacrum. It's no accident that the yoga pose that most completely exemplifies spinal flexion is called the child's pose (see figure 2.14)—it replicates the primary curve of the unborn child. From a certain perspective, all the curves of the body that are convex posteriorly can be seen as reflections of the primary curve. A simple way to identify all the primary curves is to notice all the parts of the body that contact the floor in savasana, or corpse pose (see figures 2.15 and 2.16):

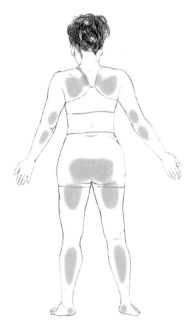

Figure 2.15 In corpse pose, the primary curves of the body contact the floor.

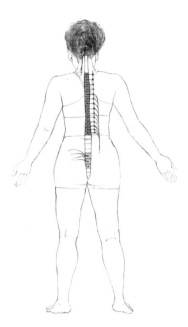

Figure 2.16   Savasana seen from below, showing spinal origins of the autonomic nervous system—sympathetic from the thoracic and parasympathetic from cervical and sacral regions.

the curve of the back of the head, the upper back, the sacrum, the backs of the thighs, the calves, and the heels. Consequently, the secondary curves are present in all the body parts that are off the floor in this position: the cervical and lumbar spine, the backs of the knees, and the space posterior to the Achilles tendons.

From this perspective, spinal flexion can be defined as an increase in the primary spinal curves and a decrease in the secondary spinal curves. A reversal of this definition would define spinal extension as an increase in the secondary curves and a decrease in the primary curves.

Note that as far as movement is concerned, the relationship between the primary and secondary curves is reciprocal: The more you increase or decrease one, the more the other will want to do the opposite. For example, an increase in thoracic kyphosis automatically produces a decrease in cervical and lumbar lordosis.

The classic yoga exercise that explores this reciprocal relationship of the primary and secondary curves is cat/cow, or chakravakasana (see figure 2.17).

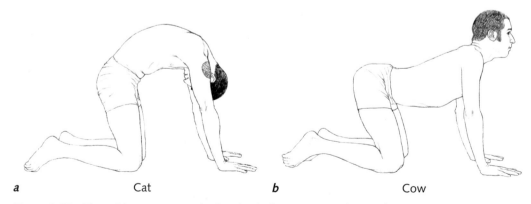

a   Cat   *b*   Cow

Figure 2.17   The cat/cow pose emphasizes both the primary and secondary curves.

Supported at both ends by the arms and thighs, the spine's curves can move freely in both directions, producing the shape changes of flexion and extension. Although it is common to teach this movement by telling the student to exhale on spinal flexion and inhale on extension, it is more accurate to say that spinal flexion *is* an exhalation and spinal extension *is* an inhalation. As the definition of breathing shows, spinal shape change is synonymous with breathing shape change (see figure 1.6 on page 6).

MOVEMENT EXPLORATION

From a comfortable sitting position, try increasing your thoracic kyphosis by dropping your chest forward. Notice how your neck and lower back flatten. Now, try the same movement, but initiate it with your head; if you drop your head forward, you'll notice how the chest and lower spine will follow. The same will occur if you initiate this movement with your lower spine. You may also notice that these flexion movements of the spine generally tend to create an exhalation.

Going in the opposite direction, try decreasing your thoracic kyphosis by lifting your chest. Notice how your neck and lower back increase their curves. If you try initiating it with your head or lower spine, the results will be the same. Did you notice how these extension movements of the spine tend to create an inhalation?

Spatial and Spinal Perspectives in Forward- and Backward-Bending Poses

Spinal extension is not necessarily the same thing as bending backward, and spinal flexion is not necessarily the same thing as bending forward. In order to avoid confusion, it's important to keep these distinctions clear. *Flexion* and *extension* refer to the relationship of the spinal curves to each other, while *forward bending* and *backward bending* are terms that refer to movements of the body in space. The terms are not interchangeable. By way of illustration, picture the following contrasting examples of how two different body types would move into and out of a standing overhead reach:

A stiff, sedentary office worker, whose stooped posture doesn't change as his hips move forward and his arms reach overhead in an attempt to do a standing backbend. His spine is remaining in flexion while his body is moving backward in space.

A flexible dancer, who hyperextends her spinal curves in the overhead reach, and keeps her spine extended as she flexes forward at the hip joints to move into uttanasana (standing forward bend). Her spine is remaining in extension while her body is bending forward in space.

The valuable skill in observing movements like this is the ability to distinguish movement of the spinal curves in relation to each other from the movements of the torso in space.

Figure 2.18 shows more of an integrated orientation to a standing backbend. Here, the secondary curves are kept under control, and the pelvis is kept firmly over the feet. As a result, there is much less movement backward in space, but a greater emphasis on thoracic extension (reduction of the primary curve). Although this is not a dramatic movement spatially, it will actually provide a safe and effective stretch to the thoracic and rib structures and will be less disturbing to the process of breathing than either the dancer's or the office worker's movements.

Spatial and Spinal Perspectives in Lateral and Twisting Movements

When looking at yoga poses that involve lateral and twisting movements, it's also important to distinguish spatial from spinal perspectives. Triangle (trikonasana) is a pose that is often referred to as a lateral stretch, and this is true insofar as it lengthens the connective tissue pathway that runs along the side of the body (see figure 2.19).

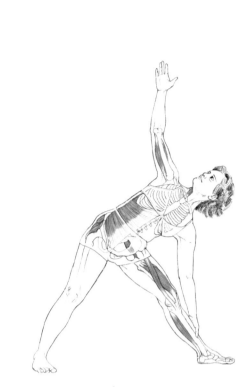

Figure 2.18   An integrated orientation to a standing backbend.

Figure 2.19   Trikonasana.

It is, however, possible to lengthen the lateral line of the body without any appreciable lateral flexion of the spine, so again, we need to be clear what exactly is meant by a term like "lateral bend."

In trikonasana, more of a lateral line stretch would result from a wide spacing of the feet, and an intention to initiate the movement primarily from the pelvis while maintaining the spine in neutral extension. This also turns the pose into more of a hip-opener.

Lateral flexion of the spine could be emphasized by a closer spacing of the feet, which allows for more stabilization of the relationship between the pelvis and thighs, which would require the movement to come from the lateral bending of the spine.

Sticking with the example of triangle pose, if we look at its revolved variation in figure 2.20, we can apply the same perspective to the twisting action of the spine. The lumbar spine is almost entirely incapable of axial rotation (only 5 degrees), which, in this pose, means that it will go wherever the sacrum leads it. Consequently, for the lower spine to twist in the direction of this pose, the pelvis would have to turn in the same direction.

If the hips are restricted, the lumbar spine will appear to be moving in the opposite direction of the rib cage and shoulder girdle rotation, and when this is the case, most of the twist will originate from first joints above the sacrum that can freely rotate: the lower thoracics, T11-T12 and above. In addition, the twisting of the shoulder girdle around the rib cage can create the illusion that the spine is twisting more than it really is. So, the body can indeed be twisting in space, but a careful observation of the spine may tell where exactly the twisting is (or is not) coming from.

If the pelvis is free to rotate around the hip joints, this pose will exhibit a more evenly distributed twist throughout the spine (rather than an overloading of T11 and T12). The

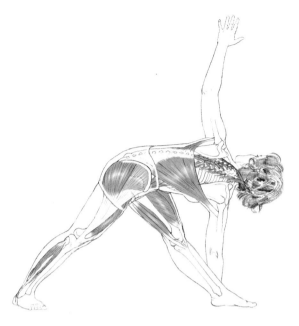

Figure 2.20   Parivrtta trikonasana.

lumbar spine will fully participate because the pelvis and sacrum are also turning; the neck and shoulders will be free, and the rib cage, upper back, and neck will be open, along with the breathing.

Axial Extension, Bandhas, and Mahamudra

Axial extension, the fifth spinal movement, is defined as a simultaneous reduction of both the primary and secondary curves of the spine (see figure 2.21). In other words, the cervical, thoracic, and lumbar curves are all reduced, and the result is that the overall length of the spine is increased.

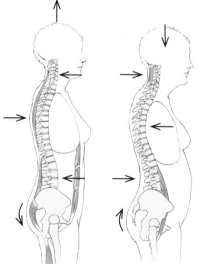

Figure 2.21   Axial extension involves a simultaneous reduction of the primary and secondary curves, which lengthens the spinal column beyond its neutral alignment.

Because the primary and secondary curves have a reciprocal relationship, which is expressed in the "natural" movements of flexion and extension, axial extension is "unnatural" in the sense that it bypasses this reciprocal relationship by reducing all three curves at once. In other words, axial extension doesn't happen all on its own; it requires conscious effort and training to accomplish.

The action that produces axial extension involves a shift in the tone and orientation of the breathing structures known as the bandhas. The three diaphragms (pelvic, respiratory, and vocal) and their surrounding musculature become more sthira (stable). As a result, the ability of the thoracic and abdominal cavities to change shape is more limited in axial extension. The overall effect is a reduction of breath volume but an increase in length.

The overall yogic term that describes this state of the spine and breath is *mahamudra*, which always involves axial extension and the bandhas. It is possible to do mahamudra from many positions, including seated, standing, supine, and in arm supports.

A seated posture named mahamudra (see figure 2.22) adds a twisting action to axial extension. It is considered a supreme accomplishment to do this practice with all three bandhas executed correctly, because it represents a complete merging of asana and pranayama practice.

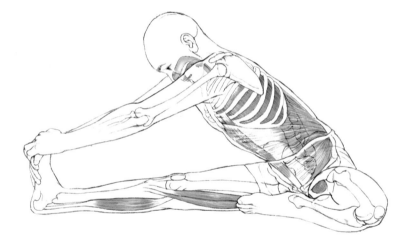

Figure 2.22   Mahamudra combines axial extension and a twisting action.

UNDERSTANDING THE ASANAS

Deciding which anatomical details of yoga poses to depict is quite a challenge. Unlike weight training and stretching, which focus on specific muscles, yoga focuses on asanas that are whole-body practices; no elements are entirely passive.[1]

Respecting the principles of yoga previously discussed, I have attempted a reconciliation of opposing imperatives in selecting the following information. I have tried to be systematic, but not formulaic, taking each posture on its own unique terms, while providing some consistency in the format of the page spreads and the information provided.

Because yoga practice is fundamentally experiential, the information in this book is intended to be an inspiration to explore your own body. Perhaps you will understand more clearly something you've experienced as a result of reviewing this material. On the other hand, some anatomical detail may capture your interest and move you to investigate it through a pose that's being depicted. In either case, this book will have served its purpose if it supports you in these explorations.

Starting Positions and the Base of Support

The poses in this book are arranged by their starting position. Every unusual position of the body has to begin with a usual position. The five "usual positions" are commonly referred to as the starting positions. Any asana you can think of has one of these common positions as its starting point:

Standing—supported on the soles of your feet (page 33)

Sitting—supported on the base of your pelvis (page 79)

Kneeling—supported on your knees, shins, and tops of feet (page 119)

Supine—supported on the back surface of your body (page 135)

Prone—supported on the front surface of your body (page 163)

Within each asana section is at least one forward bend, backbend, twist, lateral bend, and axial extension. The selections include the postures that are most commonly practiced by the majority of teaching traditions.

Related to the issue of starting position is the concept of the base of support. This refers to the parts of the body that are on the ground and through which the weight-bearing forces are transmitted down to the earth, resulting in some supporting energy generated upward into the body. Anatomically, only the feet—supporting the legs and pelvis—have evolved specifically to accomplish this. That is perhaps why the simple standing poses are considered the starting point for all asana practice by most yoga traditions. The lessons you learn from standing on the earth can be applied to any other base of support you may experience.

The structures in the body that most closely resemble the feet and legs are, of course, the hands and arms. When you employ them to create a base of support, you do arm supports, which are covered in a chapter all their own on page 175.

---

[1] Even savasana (the corpse pose), requiring complete relaxation of all the skeletal muscles, has an active component: The mind is intentionally focused on the process of breathing and relaxation—otherwise it's just napping.

Information for Each Pose

With occasional variation, each pose description includes the following sections:

- **Name.** Each asana is presented with its Sanskrit name and its translated English name. Additionally, some descriptive text is added to clarify the meaning or context of the pose's name.

- **Classification and level.** Poses are classified by their base of support, spinal action, and level of difficulty.

- **Key structures.** For each asana, at least three key structures are highlighted. These may be anatomical elements that the pose brings into greater focus or function. They could also be less obvious body parts that can provide a deeper action than you would ordinarily notice. Additionally, a particular asana description might discuss an interesting anatomical observation that could just as easily apply to several other postures.

- **Key joint and limb actions.** The joints and limbs that are involved in the asana are identified according to their actions: flexion, extension, adduction, abduction, rotation, and so forth.

- **Working and lengthening.** In the performance of any yoga asana, the most prominent sensations are generated by the lengthening and working of the skeletal muscles. Many times, muscles have to work and lengthen simultaneously to do the poses. For each pose, some element of that component is depicted and analyzed. The key muscles for each pose are discussed.

- **Breathing.** Breathing is the changing of shape of the body cavities. Each yoga posture presents a specific shape-changing challenge to the respiratory mechanism. Many postures are presented with notes on these underlying breathing patterns and suggestions on how to use the breath to get the most out of the posture's effects.

- **Obstacles and notes.** From a certain perspective, yoga is the practice of uncovering and resolving obstructions in the human system. Practicing yoga asanas is a systematic way of encountering those obstacles in the most perceptually accessible aspect of our system—the physical body. Presented are the most common obstacles to achieving each of the pictured asanas, along with some useful suggestions for overcoming them.

- **Cautions.** Certain poses present potential risk to specific body parts or to particular people. These are pointed out where applicable.

- **Variations.** For certain asanas, key variations are pictured and explained.

- **Special notes.** Here, wherever it's needed, are notes that don't fit into any of the other categories. This could include comments about the asana's terminology, history, mythology, or any other contextual information.

Types of Muscle Contractions

In the "Working and Lengthening" sections in the next chapters, four types of muscle contractions are referred to:

Concentric—The length of the muscle decreases during a contraction.

Eccentric—The length of the muscle increases during a contraction.

Isometric—The length of the muscle remains constant during a contraction against resistance, and the intention is to not move.

Isotonic—The length of the muscle remains constant during a contraction against resistance, and the intention is to move.

An understandable question that could arise is: "Since the poses are all static, why wouldn't all the muscles just be doing isometric contractions?"[2] The short answer to this question is that the text is describing how to come into a pose from a starting position, rather than how to be in a pose. In other words, look at an asanas as a *process* rather than as a final product.

Most often an image of an asana depicts the end point of a movement. Even if you stay in a pose for a period of time, the muscle actions that got you there from the starting point (standing, sitting, kneeling, and so on) are still present. In addition, the movements of the breathing structures never cease. In yoga poses, we experience a cross section of a never-ending progression of movement and breath, extending infinitely forward and backward in time.[3] As long as we are in this matrix of space and time, we will never actually be still, and our full action potential will be present and accessible.

The Drawings

The asana images in this book are based on photographs of various models that were taken during several sessions. Some of the perspectives are quite unusual, because they were shot from below using a large sheet of plexiglass, or from above using a ladder.

The photos were used as reference for the anatomical illustrator, who posed her skeleton in the various positions and sketched the bones by hand. After a round of corrections, the

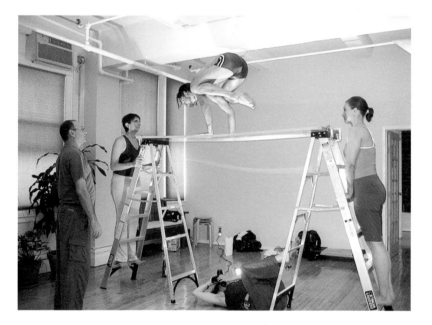

Yoga Anatomy photo shoot at The Breathing Project in New York City. Leslie Kaminoff (far left) supervises as project photographer, Lydia Mann, shoots Derek's Bakasana from below the plexiglass. Janet and Elizabeth stabilize the ladders. The final artwork from the resulting photo is on page 186.

---

[2] "Each bodily movement is embedded in a chain of infinite happenings from which we distinguish only the immediate preceding steps and, occasionally, those which immediately follow" (Laban 1966, p. 54). For reference to "isometric" versus "stabilizing isotonic," see Adler, Beckers, and Buck, 2003.

[3] A memorable description of this concept is contained in Kurt Vonnegut's *Slaughterhouse-Five*, in which he describes the Tralfamadorians, who live in the fourth dimension. When they look at a person, they see a very long, four-dimensional caterpillar, with tiny newborn legs at one end and withered, elderly legs at the other end. Human beings, lacking the fourth dimension of perception, can only see a three-dimensional cross section of the caterpillar.

muscles and other structures were added using computer software, and several more rounds of corrections and adjustments were made to produce the final images.

The labeling of the structures in each drawing, as well as the various arrows and other indicators, were added last.

When you stand, you bear weight on the only structures in the body that have specifically evolved to hold you up in the uniquely human stance—the feet. The architecture of the feet, along with their musculature, shows nature's unmatched ability to reconcile and neutralize opposing forces.

Clearly, however, these amazing structures are massively overengineered for the way most people use them in the civilized world of stiff shoes and paved surfaces. Fortunately, yoga exercises are done barefoot, with much attention given to restoring the strength and flexibility of the foot and lower leg muscles.

In yoga practice, some of the earliest lessons frequently center on the simple act of standing upright—something you've been doing (more or less successfully) since you were about a year old. If you can feel your weight releasing into the three points of contact between the foot and the earth, you may be able to feel the support that the earth gives back to you through the action of the three arches of the foot and the muscles that control them.

Standing positions have the highest center of gravity of all the starting points, and the effort of stabilizing that center makes standing poses—by definition—brahmana. Release and support, giving and receiving, inhaling and exhaling—Patanjali's formulation of sthiram sukham asanam encompasses all of these and more.[1]

The fundamental lessons you learn from standing postures can illuminate the practice of all the other asanas.

---

[1] *Patanjali's Yoga Sutra*, II.1. T.K.V. Desikachar's translation sums it up well when he defines *sthiram* as "alertness without tension" and *sukham* as "relaxation without dullness."

Tadasana

Mountain Pose

tah-DAHS-anna

tada = mountain

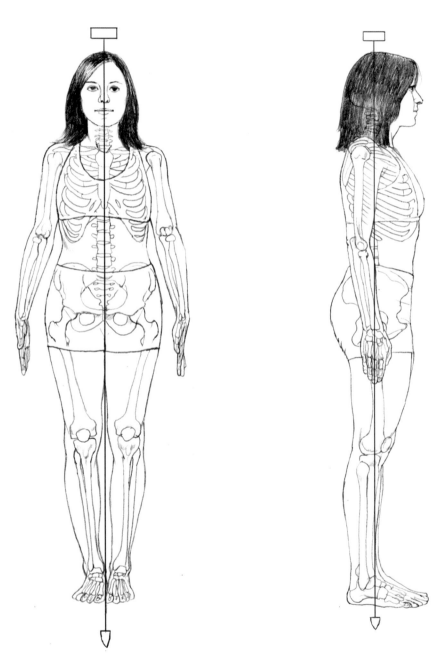

This pose's name evokes many images that relate to a stable, rooted base of support and a "crown" that reaches for the heavens.

Classification and Level

Easy standing pose

Key Structures

Intrinsic and extrinsic foot muscles, quadriceps, iliopsoas, piriformis, abdominal wall, diaphragm.

Joint Actions

The lumbar, thoracic, and cervical curves are in mild axial extension.

The ankle, hip, shoulder, and wrist joints are in their neutral positions, midway between flexion and extension.

The knee joints are extended (but not hyperextended); the elbow joints are extended and the forearms are pronated.

The arches of the feet are lifted and connecting with the upward lifting action in the pelvic floor, the lower abdomen, rib cage, cervical spine, and the top of the head.

The shoulder blades are dropped onto the support of the rib cage and connect with the downward release of the tailbone and the grounding of the three points of contact between each foot and the floor.

Notes

Nothing lasting can be built on a shaky foundation. This may be why tadasana is considered by many yoga traditions to be the starting point of asana practice. Interestingly, this pose is almost identical to the "anatomical position"—the starting reference point for the study of movement and anatomy. The only major difference between the two positions is that in tadasana, the palms of the hands are facing the sides of the thighs rather than forward.

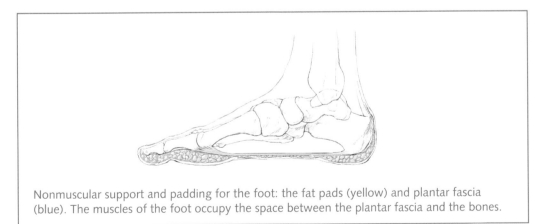

Nonmuscular support and padding for the foot: the fat pads (yellow) and plantar fascia (blue). The muscles of the foot occupy the space between the plantar fascia and the bones.

(continued)

Tadasana   *(continued)*

This body position is also uniquely human, because humans are the only true biped mammals on the planet. Humans are also the least stable of creatures, possessing the smallest base of support, the highest center of gravity, and (proportionately) the heaviest brain balancing atop it all.

The base of support of this pose—the feet—offers a beautiful image of how the passive and active forces of release and support operate in the human system. The essential structure of the foot can be represented by a triangle. The three points of the triangle are the three places where the foot's structure will rest on a supporting surface: the calcaneal tuberosity, the base of the first metatarsal, and the base of the fifth metatarsal. The lines connecting these points represent the arches—three lines of lift through which postural support is derived: the medial longitudinal arch, the lateral longitudinal arch, and the transverse (metatarsal) arch.

From underneath, the two triangles of the feet can be joined to show the size and shape of the base of support for tadasana. The "plumb line" that passes through the body's center of gravity in this position should also fall through the exact center of this base.

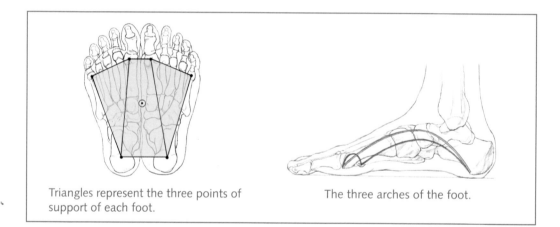

Triangles represent the three points of support of each foot.

The three arches of the foot.

The four layers of musculature (see top figure on page 37) all combine to create lift, balance, and movement of the 28 bones of the foot, which has evolved to be an incredibly adaptable structure able to move you smoothly through space over uneven terrain.

The foot has evolved over millions of years in a world with no roads or sidewalks. In today's world in which many uneven surfaces have been leveled and paved, it's clearly overengineered. When the adaptability of the foot is no longer needed for locomotion, the deeper muscles that support the arches inevitably weaken, eventually leaving only the superficial, noncontractile plantar fascia responsible for preventing the total collapse of the foot. This frequently leads to plantar fasciitis and heel spurs.

The practice of standing postures in general, and tadasana in particular, is one of the best ways to restore the natural aliveness, strength, and adaptability of the feet. Once your foundation is improved, it's much easier to put the rest of your house in order.

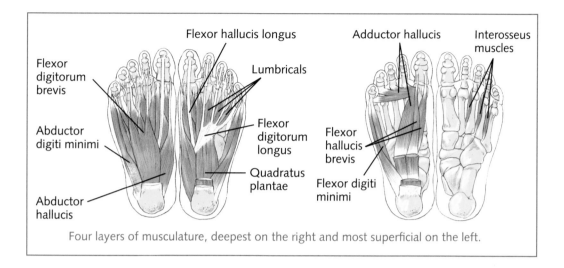

Four layers of musculature, deepest on the right and most superficial on the left.

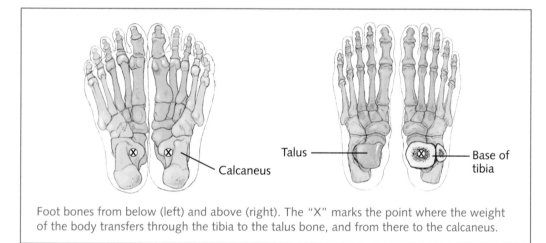

Foot bones from below (left) and above (right). The "X" marks the point where the weight of the body transfers through the tibia to the talus bone, and from there to the calcaneus.

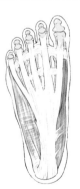

The plantar fascia—the most superficial layer of support for the foot. The more the arch support muscles weaken, the more pressure is put on the plantar fascia, which can result in plantar fasciitis and heel spurs.

(continued)

Tadasana   *(continued)*

Tadasana Variation

Samasthiti

Equal Standing, Prayer Pose
   sama = same, equal
   sthiti = to establish, to stand

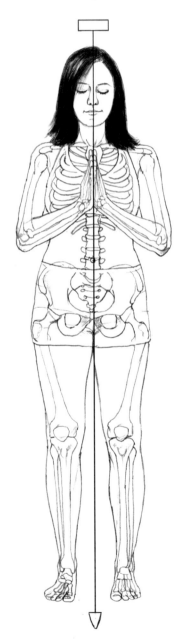
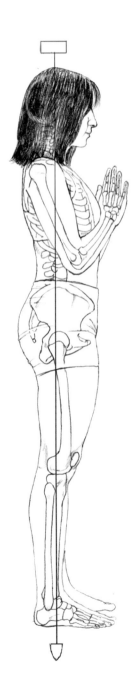

Samasthiti has a wider, more stable base than tadasana because the feet are placed with the heels under the sitting bones rather than touching each other. All the standing poses that are executed from this base, as opposed to tadasana, consequently have a wider, more stable base of support. This is typically done in the vinyasa styles, in which breath-coordinated movement is the focus, rather than the alignment-oriented approaches, in which static maintenance of positions is preferred.

Additionally, the head is lowered and the hands are in namaste (prayer) position. This is typical of the starting point of a sun salutation, a prayerful vinyasa that is used by many systems of hatha yoga as a warm-up and to connect asanas into a flowing sequence.

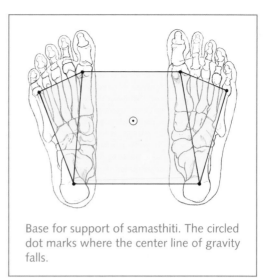

Base for support of samasthiti. The circled dot marks where the center line of gravity falls.

Terminology Note

In the Ashtanga tradition of Sri K. Pattabhi Jois, the term *samasthiti* refers to what is here described as tadasana. In the teaching tradition of Sri T. Krishnamacharya and his son, T.K.V. Desikachar, the term *tadasana* refers to a standing pose with the arms overhead, and balancing on the balls of the feet.

Cautions

People with headache, insomnia, and low blood pressure should exercise caution when performing prolonged standing poses.

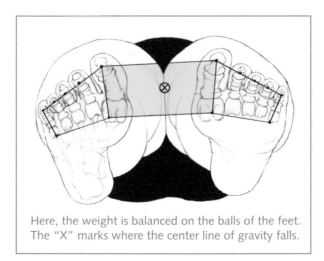

Here, the weight is balanced on the balls of the feet. The "X" marks where the center line of gravity falls.

Utkatasana

Chair Pose

OOT-kah-TAHS-anna

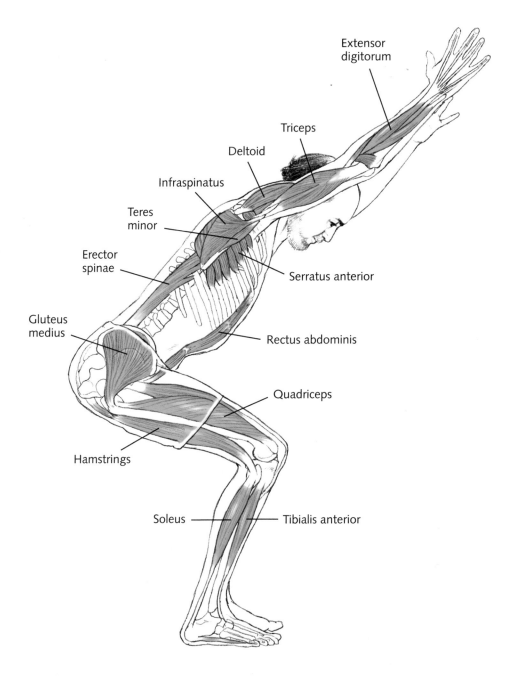

Extensor digitorum

Triceps

Deltoid

Infraspinatus

Teres minor

Erector spinae

Serratus anterior

Gluteus medius

Rectus abdominis

Quadriceps

Hamstrings

Soleus

Tibialis anterior

Classification and Level

Basic standing pose, axial extension

Key Structures

Shoulder girdle, spine, quadriceps and hamstrings to balance each other, knees (adductors and medial rotators). To protect knees, minimize external rotation as the hips flex.

Joint Actions

Shoulder flexion, elbow extension, forearm supination, axial extension in spine, hip and knee flexion, ankle dorsiflexion.

Working

Spine: Intertransversarii, interspinalis, transversospinalis group, erector spinae, psoas minor.

Shoulders and arms: Upper trapezius, serratus anterior, supraspinatus, middle deltoids, biceps brachii long head, triceps, supinator, extensor digitorum, abdominal muscles (to maintain axial extension and support lower spine).

Legs: Gluteus medius and minimus, adductor group, quadriceps eccentrically (modulated and balanced by hamstrings), tibialis anterior, soleus eccentrically, intrinsic muscles of the feet.

Lengthening

Latissimus dorsi, rhomboids, gluteus maximus, soleus.

Breathing

Maintaining axial extension (which minimizes breathing shape change) while engaging the largest, most oxygen-hungry muscles of the body presents a challenge that requires efficiency of effort and breath. Otherwise, the body's oxygen demands will make the breath too labored to continue to maintain the axial extension.

Obstacles

Tight latissimus dorsi, weak quadriceps, knees falling out of alignment, over-arching lumbar spine (hence, psoas minor and abdominal muscles), over-flexing hips (hence, hamstrings, to resist the quadriceps' tendency to pull the sitting bones away from the backs of the knees).

Notes

Knees are vulnerable in this position (partly flexed), particularly the menisci, if there is excessive knee rotation.

Gravity should be the main source of resistance in the pose, not the resistance of agonist and antagonist contraction. Beginning students in this asana tend to feel a lot heavier than their weight because of this.

Uttanasana

Standing Forward Bend

OOT-tan-AHS-anna

ut = intense

tan = stretch

Classification and Level

Easy standing pose, forward bend

Key Structures

Hip joint, legs, spine.

Joint Actions

Hip flexion, knee extension, mild spinal flexion (the tighter the hamstrings, the more the spinal flexion).

Working

Upper body: Gravity.

Lower body: Vastus medialis, intermedius, lateralis (knee extensors); articularis genus (to draw up on the capsule of the knee joint); feet and ankles (for balance).

Lengthening

Spinal muscles, hamstrings, posterior fibers of gluteus medius and minimus, gluteus maximus, piriformis, adductor magnus, soleus, gastrocnemius.

Breathing

Deep hip flexion compresses the abdomen. This combined with gravity moves the center of the diaphragm cranially, so more freedom is needed in the back of the rib cage for the movement of the breath.

Piriformis

Spinal extensors

Hamstrings

Gastrocnemius

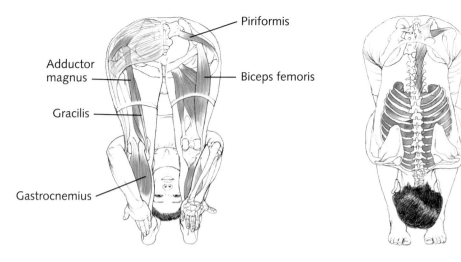

Obstacles

Tightness in hamstrings, spinal muscles, gluteals.

Cautions

People with back injury, osteoporosis, or both should approach deep forward bending very cautiously and gradually.

People with high blood pressure (hypertension) should go into this pose gradually and remain in it only if their breathing is not strained. People with low blood pressure (hypotension) should come out of this pose very slowly, because they may become dizzy.

Notes

In this pose, gravity should do the work. People experiencing tightness in the back of the legs sometimes pull themselves down, which creates tightness and congestion in the rectus femoris and psoas. It's better to soften the knees to find some space in the hip joint, allowing the spine to release. Only then does lengthening the legs produce an even stretch along the entire back line of the body.

For more anatomy, and the seated version of this pose, see paschimottanasana, page 82.

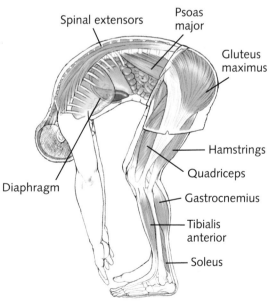

If the hamstrings are tight, slightly bending the knees helps release the spine.

Utthita Hasta Padangusthasana

Extended Hand–Toe Pose or Standing Big Toe Hold

oo-TEE-tah HA-sta pad-an goosh-TAHS-anna

utthita = extended

hasta = hand

pada = foot

angusta = big toe

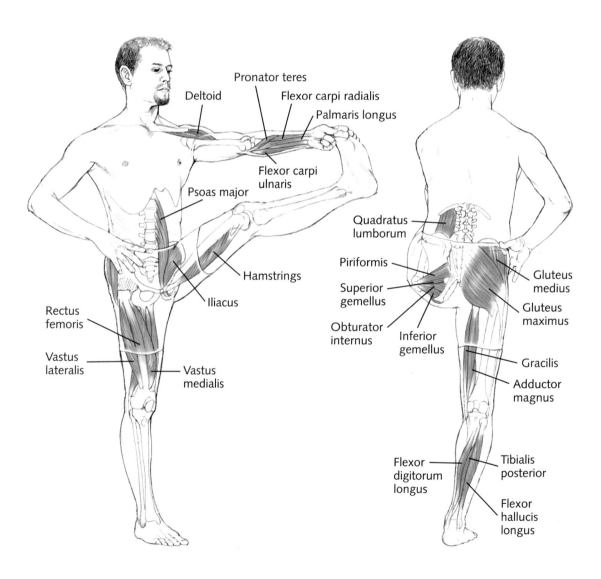

Deltoid

Pronator teres

Flexor carpi radialis

Palmaris longus

Flexor carpi ulnaris

Psoas major

Hamstrings

Iliacus

Rectus femoris

Vastus lateralis

Vastus medialis

Quadratus lumborum

Piriformis

Superior gemellus

Obturator internus

Inferior gemellus

Gluteus medius

Gluteus maximus

Gracilis

Adductor magnus

Flexor digitorum longus

Tibialis posterior

Flexor hallucis longus

Classification and Level

Intermediate asymmetrical standing balance pose

Joint Actions

Neutral spine, pelvis level, shoulder flexion, elbow extension, finger flexion. Standing leg: neutral hip extension, knee extension (not locked). Lifted leg: hip flexion, knee extension.

Working

Standing leg, spine, and pelvis: Quadriceps and hamstrings on the standing leg; spinal extensors, to keep from flexing the spine and tucking the pelvis; abductors and external rotators, eccentrically, to keep the pelvis level; external and internal obliques; rotary muscles of the back (obliques, transversospinalis), to counter the rotation created by the arm holding the toe.

Lifted leg: Flexors of the shoulder and fingers to hold the big toe and create hip flexion; psoas major and iliacus, rectus femoris, pectineus, adductor brevis and longus (to help with hip flexion).

Lengthening

Lifted leg: Hamstrings, gastrocnemius, soleus, gluteus maximus.

Obstacles

Tightness in the hamstrings or gluteus maximus in the lifted leg can cause spinal flexion, and thus hip extension or knee flexion in the standing leg. It's better to bend the knee in the lifted leg and find neutral curves in the spine and neutral extension in the standing hip, and knee extension (but not hyperextension) in the standing leg.

Notes

Weakness in standing leg abductors can create "hip hike" on the side of the lifted leg, leading to overwork of the quadratus lumborum.

Weakness in the hip flexors (psoas major, iliacus, and rectus femoris) can also cause overwork in the quadratus lumborum and hip hike.

Breathing

In maintaining this balance pose, the stabilizing action in the abdominal muscles combines with the bracing action of the arms to create an overall reduction of breathing capacity. If there is excessive muscular tension, the reduced volume of breath will not be sufficient to fuel the effort, and the increased volume of breath will tend to compromise the balance.

Vrksasana

Tree Pose

vrik-SHAHS-anna

vrksa = tree

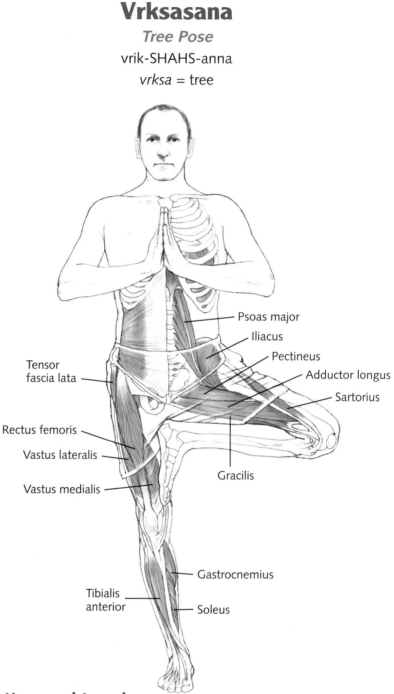

Psoas major

Iliacus

Pectineus

Adductor longus

Sartorius

Tensor fascia lata

Rectus femoris

Vastus lateralis

Vastus medialis

Gracilis

Gastrocnemius

Tibialis anterior

Soleus

Classification and Level

Basic asymmetrical standing balance

Key Structures

Lower leg, foot, arch, abductors, and external rotators of the standing leg; external and internal obliques, to stabilize torso to pelvis.

Joint and Limb Actions

Neutral spine, level pelvis. Standing leg: hip neutral extension, internal rotation, adduction; knee extension (not locked). Lifted leg: hip flexion, external rotation, abduction; knee flexion; tibia external rotation; ankle dorsiflexion (pressed against the adductors of the standing leg); foot pronation.

Working

Lifted leg: Iliacus and psoas major, all external rotators and extensors—gluteus maximus, posterior fibers of gluteus medius and minimus, piriformis, adductor magnus (extensor portion), obturator internus and externus, gemelli, quadratus femoris.

Standing leg: Piriformis, tensor fascia lata, gluteus medius and minimus, gluteus maximus (extensor portion).

Standing foot: Intrinsic muscles of the foot, muscles of the ankle and lower leg.

Lengthening

Lifted leg: Pectineus, adductor longus and brevis, gracilis.

Standing leg: Gluteus medius and minimus, piriformis (working eccentrically).

Notes

The adductors lengthen to get into position; they may have some role in holding the leg in place by pressing the foot into the inside of the standing leg. Misusing the pectineus to hold the leg in place creates flexion at the hip, tilting the pelvis and rotating the leg inward.

Abductors on the standing leg are working eccentrically; if they are weak or tight, the hip of the lifted leg will "hike up," or the rotators will try to stabilize the pelvis and the pelvis will rotate open.

The more strength and adaptability you have in the feet and ankles, the more options you will have for finding balance.

Breathing

Compared to tree pose with arms elevated (next variation) or utthita hasta padangusthasana (the toe-hold posture), the upper body is freer to participate in respiratory movements in this pose. With the arms held quietly in namaste, and the raised leg braced against the adductors of the standing leg, the attention and center of gravity are drawn inward and downward.

Cautions

People with inner ear or balance disorders (benign positional vertigo, Ménière's disease) should practice standing balances near a wall for extra security and support.

(continued)

Vrksasana Variation

Tree Pose With Arms Elevated

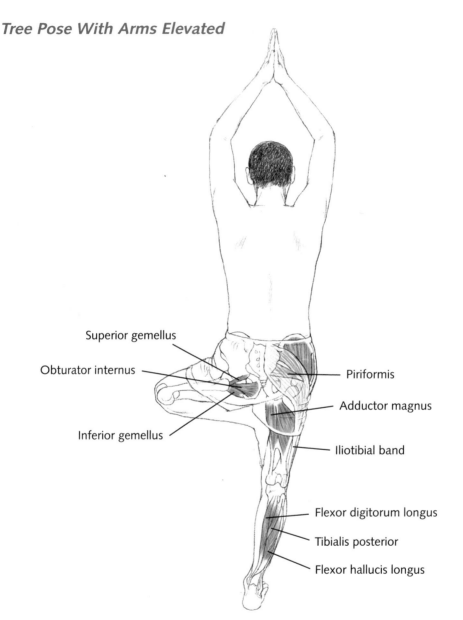

Superior gemellus

Obturator internus

Piriformis

Adductor magnus

Inferior gemellus

Iliotibial band

Flexor digitorum longus

Tibialis posterior

Flexor hallucis longus

Classification and Level

Intermediate asymmetrical standing balance pose

Joint Actions

Neutral spine; scapula upward rotation, abduction, elevation; glenohumeral external rotation, abduction; elbow extension; forearm pronation (if the upper arm is externally rotated).

Working

Infraspinatus, teres minor, deltoids, supraspinatus, long head biceps, serratus anterior (supported by the upper fibers of the trapezius), triceps with anconeus to extend elbows.

Lengthening

Latissimus dorsi, teres major, long head triceps.

Obstacles and Notes

Overuse of the latissimus dorsi to "pull shoulders down the back" interferes with the elevation of the scapulae; it can create impingement at the acromion of the biceps tendon and supraspinatus. The rib cage can also be pushed forward from a restriction of the latissimus.

This variation creates a higher center of gravity by placing the arms overhead, and is therefore categorized as an intermediate-level balancing asana.

Breathing

Because of the stabilizing action of the muscles that keep the arms overhead, the thoracic movements of the breath encounter more resistance in this position. In addition, the higher center of gravity will tend to produce a stronger stabilizing action in the abdominal muscles. Taken together, these factors combine to reduce the overall excursion of the diaphragm; therefore, quiet, efficient breathing is the most appropriate pattern. Breaths that are too deep will destabilize the posture.

Garudasana

Eagle Pose

gah-rue-DAHS-anna

garuda = a fierce bird of prey, the vehicle (vahana) of the Hindu god Vishnu, usually described as an eagle, but sometimes as a hawk or kite

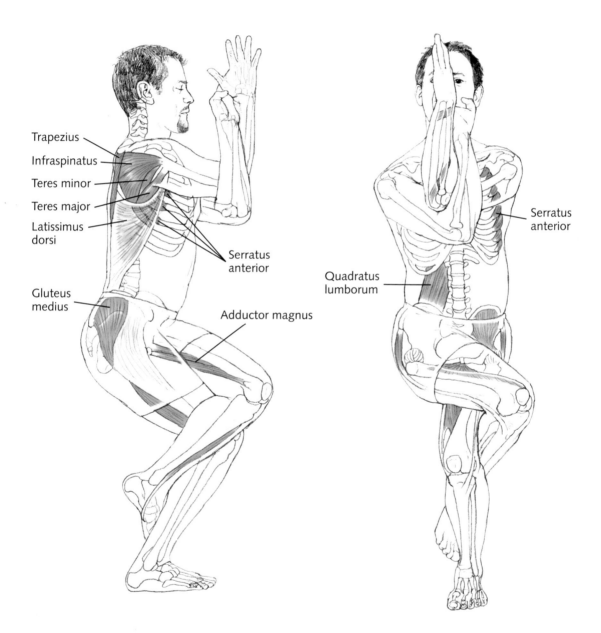

Trapezius

Infraspinatus

Teres minor

Teres major

Latissimus dorsi

Serratus anterior

Gluteus medius

Adductor magnus

Serratus anterior

Quadratus lumborum

Classification and Level

Asymmetrical standing balancing pose

Joint Actions

Mild spinal flexion; scapula abduction, upward and lateral rotation, elevation; glenohumeral external rotation; elbow flexion; forearm pronation; neutral wrist extension; pelvis anterior tilt, counternutation; hip flexion, internal rotation, adduction; knee flexion, internal rotation; ankle dorsiflexion; foot—lifted in eversion, standing in slight supination.

Working

Arm position: Infraspinatus (both working and lengthening), serratus anterior, pectoralis major and minor, coracobrachialis, pronator teres and pronator quadratus.

Leg position: Gluteus medius and minimus (anterior fibers), tensor fascia latae, adductor magnus, gluteus medius and minimus also working to stabilize the standing hip.

Lengthening

Arm position: Because of the abduction of the scapulae—rhomboids, lower trapezius, teres major, and latissimus dorsi (slightly); infraspinatus, triceps (slightly).

Leg position: Gluteus maximus, piriformis, quadratus femoris, obturator internus, posterior fibers of gluteus medius and minimus.

Obstacles and Notes

The scapulae need to be able to both abduct and rotate laterally. If the scapulae are too "pulled down," the spine will have to contort to achieve the entwined position.

Both the standing and the lifted leg need to internally rotate and adduct in this position.

To achieve the full entwining, the standing leg needs to flex at the hip and knee. This position of hip flexion with internal rotation and adduction is not structurally easy (the fibers of the hip joint capsule make it easier to internally rotate when the hip is in extension). The adduction with internal rotation especially gets to the piriformis. This position can be overmobilizing for the knees; if the hips are too tight to achieve the actions, the knees can be forced to overrotate. This action is stabilizing for the sacroiliac joint.

Breathing

This is the most "compacted" of the one-legged balancing postures, from the standpoint of both the shape and center of gravity, and the breathing. The entwining of the arms compresses the rib cage, and the hip flexion, combined with the mild spinal flexion, compresses the lower abdomen.

Natarajasana

King of the Dancers Pose

not-ah-raj-AHS-anna

nata = dancer

raja = king

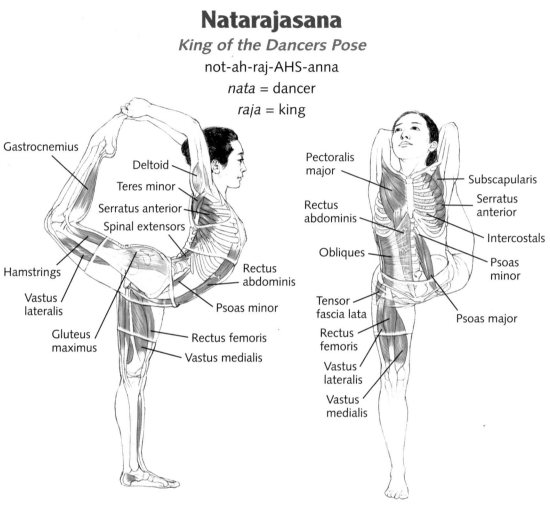

Classification and Level

Advanced backbending standing balance

Joint Actions

Spinal extension; scapula upward rotation, abduction, and elevation; arm flexion; elbow flexion; and forearm supination. Standing leg: hip flexion, knee extension, and ankle dorsiflexion. Lifted leg: hip extension, knee flexion, and ankle plantarflexion.

Working

Arms: The serratus anterior works to wrap the scapula around the rib cage; the infraspinatus and teres minor externally rotate the glenohumeral joint; and the deltoids lift the arms into position. The supraspinatus and subscapularis are also active to help hold the head of the humerus in its socket.

Spine: The intrinsic extensor muscles of the spine—intertransversarii, interspinalis, rotatores, multifidi, spinalis, semispinalis, splenius capitis and cervicis, longissimus, and iliocostalis—are all active in creating and maintaining spinal extension. The psoas minor, rectus abdominis, and obliques should all work eccentrically against the action of the spinal extensors to prevent too much action in the lumbar spine, and move more action into thoracic spinal extension and hip extension.

Standing leg: The gluteus medius and minimus and the tensor fascia latae work eccentrically to keep the pelvis level. The quadriceps extend the knee, and the hamstrings lengthen (if there's enough range of motion in the hamstrings, they might work eccentrically to resist tipping too far forward). The muscles of the feet and forelegs are active for balance.

Lifted leg: The hamstrings create hip extension and knee flexion, and the vastii come into isometric or concentric action as knee extensors as the pose deepens, to increase the hip extension against the resistance of the hand on the foot. The adductor magnus is active as both an adductor and hip extensor, and the gluteus maximus (though not as an external rotator).

Lengthening

Arms: Rhomboids, latissimus dorsi, triceps, pectoralis major.

Spine: Rectus abdominis, obliques, intercostals.

Standing leg: Hamstrings, abductors (working eccentrically).

Lifted leg: Iliacus, psoas major, rectus femoris.

Obstacles and Notes

Scapula mobility is important in this "full-arm" version—both for getting the arm into position without overmobilizing the glenohumeral joint and for mobility in the thoracic spine.

Find the deeper, more intrinsic back muscles to do the action of spinal extension. Using the latissimus and other superficial back muscles will interfere with breathing and with the ability to find the full range of motion in the scapulae.

It is also a challenge to keep the legs adducted and internally rotated in this action. Although many people seek more extension through external rotation, this involves the risk of overmobilizing the sacroiliac joint or overworking the lumbar spine.

As in dhanurasana, the binding of the hands and feet can put pressure into vulnerable spots such as the knees and lower back.

Breathing

The excursion of the diaphragm is greatly minimized in dancer's pose by the combination of deep spinal extension and the anterior and posterior musculature working against each other to stabilize this shape in gravity. Consequently, this pose should be held with quiet breathing, and seldom for a very long time, because the muscular effort required to maintain it soon outpaces the body's ability to supply those muscles with oxygen. The longer the pose is held, the deeper the body will need to breathe, and the more the abdominal muscles and the diaphragm will release their stabilizing actions, leading to an increased risk to the spine and shoulders.

Virabhadrasana I

Warrior I

veer-ah-bah-DRAHS-anna

virabhadra = the name of a fierce mythical warrior

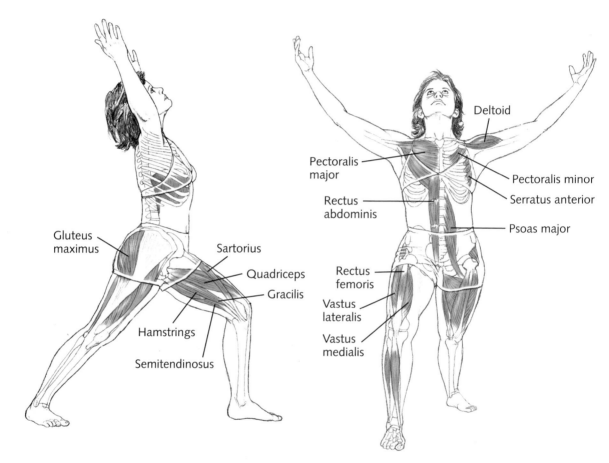

Classification and Level

Basic asymmetrical standing backbend

Key Structures

Articulate pelvis, integrity of spine, action in legs (rotation to balance the pelvis).

Joint Actions

Spinal extension; shoulder flexion, slight abduction of scapulae. Front leg: nutation, hip flexion, knee flexion, ankle dorsiflexion. Back leg: counternutation, hip extension (internal rotation), knee extension, ankle dorsiflexion and supination (to keep the heel grounded and the arch lifted).

Working

Spinal extensors, serratus anterior, deltoids, teres minor, infraspinatus, rectus abdominis (eccentrically), left internal obliques and right external obliques, psoas minor, anterior neck (rectus capitis, longus capitis, longus colli, verticalis, scalenes [eccentrically]). Front leg: hamstrings and quadriceps, eccentrically. Back leg: hamstrings and quadriceps, concentrically.

Lengthening

Latissimus dorsi, rectus abdominis, pectoralis major and minor, anterior neck (rectus capitis, longus capitis, longus colli, verticalis, scalenes). Front leg: hamstrings and quadriceps, slightly. Back leg: rectus femoris, vastii, psoas major, iliacus, soleus, and gastrocnemius.

Obstacles

Tight latissimus can pull the spine into too much of a lumbar curve.

Balance Issues

Severe sacroiliac instability, although this pose is used to improve sacroiliac problems that may arise from too much prolonged seated practice.

Notes

The shorter (from front to back) and wider (from side to side) stance of this basic warrior pose employs an easier action in the pelvis and a higher center of gravity, but it is generally an easier pose to balance in because of the wider base of support and the increased freedom of the hip joints.

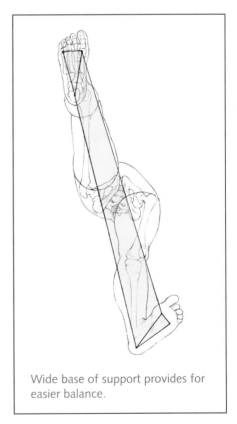

Wide base of support provides for easier balance.

(continued)

Breathing

In all the warrior poses, positioning and maintaining the pelvis' relationship to the legs and torso requires strong action in the abdominal wall, which reduces the downward excursion of the central tendon of the diaphragm. As a result, the contraction of the diaphragm will have more of a tendency to create a brahmana effect by lifting upward the base of the rib cage—an action that will only occur efficiently if there is not undue tension in the intercostals, chest, and neck muscles.

In short, the challenging leg, pelvis, and arm positions of the warrior poses combine to create interesting challenges to the breath mechanics.

Variation

Extended Warrior I

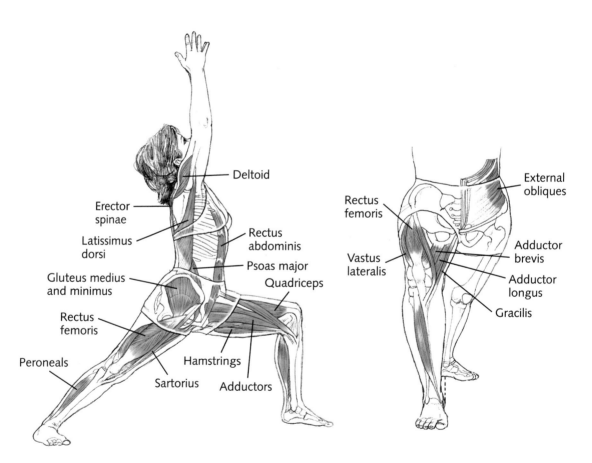

Classification and Level

Intermediate asymmetrical standing backbend

Joint Actions

Same as basic warrior but with deeper lumbar extension against anterior tilt of pelvis, adduction of legs, more supination in back foot, adduction of arms, more rotation in spine.

Working

Spinal extensors (intrinsics, transverso-spinalis, erector spinae), anterior and middle deltoids, serratus anterior, pectoralis major and minor, upper trapezius, rectus abdominis. Front leg: hamstrings eccentrically, adductors, gluteus medius and minimus. Back leg: hamstrings concentrically, gluteus medius and minimus, peroneals, quadriceps, sartorius.

Lengthening

Latissimus dorsi, rhomboids, rectus abdominis, external obliques. Front leg: quadriceps (at knee joint), hamstrings (at hip joint), gluteus medius and minimus. Back leg: peroneals, gluteus medius and minimus, psoas major, rectus femoris (at hip joint).

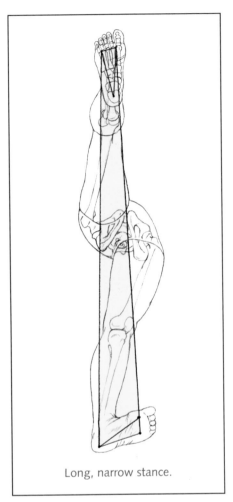

Long, narrow stance.

Obstacles

Tightness in psoas major and rectus femoris.

Weakness in hamstrings.

Weakness in eccentric control of abductors (for balance) and quadriceps in the front leg.

Notes

If the latissimus dorsi are used to do the spinal extension necessary in this deeper action, they will interfere with the lifting and lateral rotation of the arms.

A long, narrow stance is a more challenging action in the pelvis, works the abductors to balance, and provides a lower center of gravity (i.e., can be easier to balance).

Breathing

This variation of the warrior is used mostly when the pose is done statically, with no vinyasa (dynamic movement into and out of an asana). The hips and groin need to be quite open, and the legs must be strong for the breathing to be comfortable in this deeply lunged position. If the lower body can't provide effective support (sthira) for the upper body, there won't be enough freedom (sukha) for easy breathing.

Virabhadrasana II

Warrior II

veer-ah-bah-DRAHS-anna

virabhadra = the name of a fierce mythical warrior

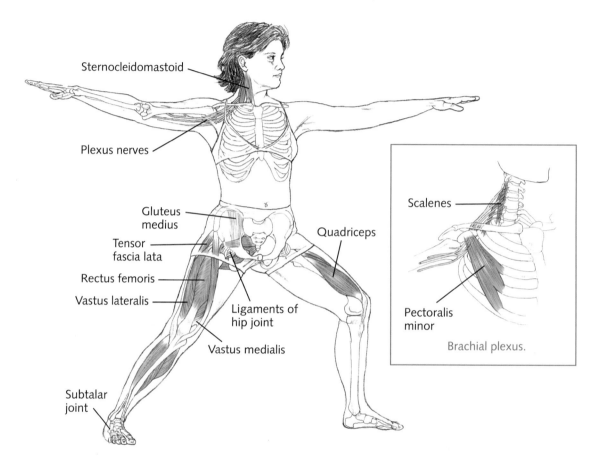

Sternocleidomastoid

Plexus nerves

Gluteus medius

Tensor fascia lata

Rectus femoris

Vastus lateralis

Ligaments of hip joint

Vastus medialis

Subtalar joint

Quadriceps

Scalenes

Pectoralis minor

Brachial plexus.

Classification and Level

Basic asymmetrical standing hip opener

Joint Actions

Spine in neutral extension; head rotated on axis; scapula upward rotation; upper arm abduction, external rotation; forearm pronation (opposing spirals in arms).

Front leg: Nutation; hip flexion, external rotation, abduction; knee flexion; ankle dorsiflexion.

Back leg: Counternutation; hip extension, internal rotation, abduction; knee extension, external rotation at tibia; ankle dorsiflexion; foot supination at heel, pronation at forefoot (arch lifted, big toe grounded).

Working

Back hip joint: Primarily gluteus medius and minimus, for internal rotation and abduction; gluteus maximus and hamstrings, for extension; tensor fascia latae, for internal rotation; pectineus for internal rotation; vastii, to extend knee.

Front hip joint: Hamstrings and quadriceps (eccentrically), gluteus maximus, piriformis, obturator internus and externus, quadratus femoris, gemelli, gluteus medius and minimus (posterior fibers).

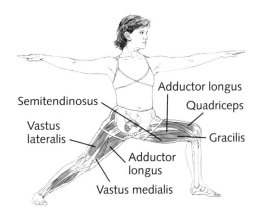

Virabhadrasana II extended.

Lengthening

Back hip joint: Tensor fascia lata, iliopsoas.

Front hip joint: Hamstrings and quadriceps (vastii).

Obstacles and Notes

Back hip joint: Abduction and extension at the same time is a challenging position for the ligaments and capsule of the hip joint. The work of the abductors (gluteus medius and minimus) is important; they help to lift the back knee away from the floor. If the gluteus medius and minimus are weak or tight, other muscles will be recruited, but they will also bring in external rotation or flexion at the hip, which will show up as an inability to "ground" the back foot.

Back ankle joint: Articulation is needed in the subtalar joint and the joints between the tarsals and metatarsals: The back part of the foot supinates so the calcaneus can clearly connect to the floor, and the forefoot pronates so the toes can clearly connect to the floor. If the foot doesn't articulate in this way, the outer ankle can be overstretched and weakened.

Front hip joint: In this position, gravity creates the flexion at the knee and hip; the hamstrings and quadriceps are very active eccentrically to modulate the pull of gravity. As with warrior I, different arrangements of the feet will affect the challenges of this pose. The more extended stance creates deeper actions at all the joints of the lower extremities, but without sufficient muscular strength in the legs (which can be developed by working in the "basic" stance), stress can be placed on the joints and connective tissues.

Breathing

See page 56.

Virabhadrasana III

Warrior III

veer-ah-bah-DRAHS-anna

virabhadra = the name of a fierce mythical warrior

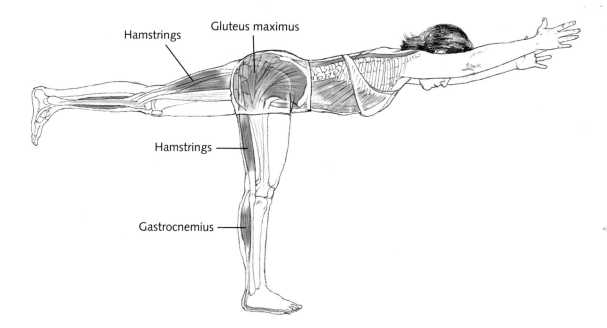

Hamstrings

Gluteus maximus

Hamstrings

Gastrocnemius

Classification and Level

Intermediate asymmetrical standing balance

Joint Actions

Spine axial extension, shoulder flexion and lateral rotation, elbow extension, forearm supination, finger extension. Front leg: nutation, hip flexion and adduction, knee extension, and ankle dorsiflexion. Back leg: counternutation, hip neutral extension and medial rotation, knee extension, ankle dorsiflexion.

Working

Spinal extensors against gravity, abdominal muscles and psoas minor to maintain a neutral spine. Both legs' hamstrings: standing leg eccentrically, back leg concentrically against gravity. Standing leg abductors: eccentrically to maintain level pelvis; standing leg gluteus maximus, deep rotators eccentrically to maintain level pelvis.

Lengthening

Standing leg hamstrings, standing leg abductors, gluteus maximus, deep external rotators.

Obstacles

Weakness in spinal and abdominal muscles.

Tight hamstrings, especially medial.

Tight or weak abductors and rotators (need to be strong in a long position).

Overusing the gluteus maximus will externally rotate either or both legs.

Notes

The spine is in axial extension; the work is to maintain the spinal curves in this relationship to gravity, balancing the abdominal action with the back extensors. If abdominal support is lacking, the extensors will overwork, and the spine will arch excessively.

Gravity draws the unsupported side of the pelvis toward the floor. Generally you don't need to use the adductors to do this; instead, the ability of the abductors and external rotators to lengthen with control is essential (otherwise the pelvis is lifted away from floor).

If hamstrings are tight, bending the standing leg is better than rotating the pelvis.

Breathing

The bandhas (see page 16) create the axial extension that supports the torso in this pose, and by definition, that reduces the overall volume of the breath. Ujjayi breathing is an important ingredient in this process.

Utthita Parsvakonasana

Extended Side Angle Pose

oo-TEE-tah parsh-vah-cone-AHS-anna

utthita = extended

parsva = side, flank

kona = angle

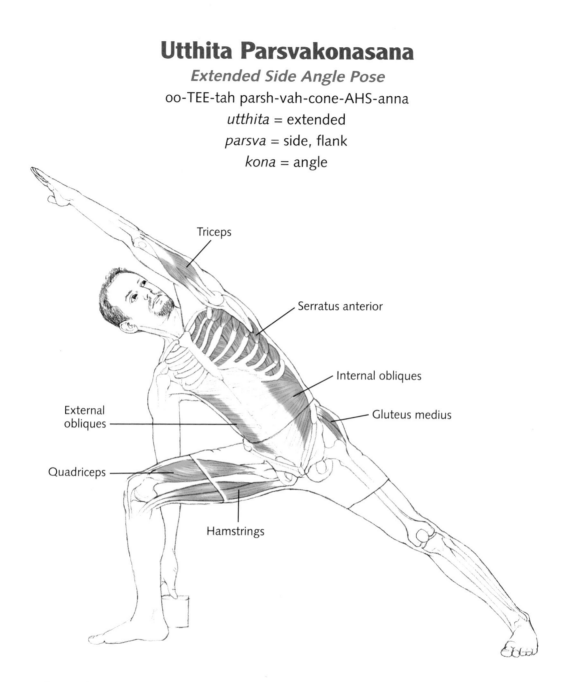

Triceps

Serratus anterior

Internal obliques

External obliques

Gluteus medius

Quadriceps

Hamstrings

Classification and Level

Basic lateral stretching, asymmetrical standing pose

Joint Actions

Spine neutral or with slight lateral flexion; shoulder abduction, upward rotation; glenohumeral joint flexion and external rotation; elbow extension. Front leg: nutation; hip flexion, external rotation, abduction; knee flexion;

ankle dorsiflexion. Back leg: counternutation; hip extension, internal rotation, abduction; knee extension (external rotation at tibia); ankle dorsiflexion; foot supination at heel; pronation at forefoot.

Working

Front leg (compare to virabhadrasana II): With increased hip flexion, the eccentric action of the hamstrings and vastii become more important—the hamstrings because they are resisting the weight of the spine over the front leg and are working at greater length, and the vastii because the rectus femoris is shortened and less effective with greater hip flexion.

Upper side (arm, spine, and back leg): Serratus anterior, deltoids, triceps, lower side external obliques, upper side internal obliques. In the back leg, the action is similar to virabhadrasana II: primarily gluteus medius and minimus (the anterior fibers help with internal rotation, the posterior fibers with abduction); gluteus maximus, for extension (but not external rotation); tensor fascia lata, for internal rotation (but not flexion); pectineus for internal rotation (but not flexion); hamstrings (more semimembranosus); quadriceps to extend the knee (more vastii than rectus femoris).

Notes

In the front leg, the increased hip flexion makes it more challenging to maintain abduction and external rotation in the leg, which keeps the knee from falling inward or the hip from swinging out.

The increased hip flexion does make it possible for the lower side of the body to stay long and for the spine to maintain its neutral length. If there is not enough hip flexion, the spine will flex laterally.

The upper arm, spine, and back leg form one continuous diagonal line. It can be a challenge to keep the spine in line with the leg in this position and not to flex in the back hip joint.

Breathing

Even though the upper side of the breathing mechanism receives a strong stretch in this shape, the more interesting effect may be on the lower side of the body, where the dome of the diaphragm is driven cranially by the force of gravity acting on the abdominal organs. Breath action in this position provides very useful asymmetrical stimulation to the diaphragm and all the organs attaching to it.

Parivrtta Baddha Parsvakonasana

Revolved Side Angle Pose

par-ee-vrt-tah BAH-dah parsh-vah-cone-AHS-anna

parivrtta = twist, revolve

baddha = bound

parsva = side, flank

kona = angle

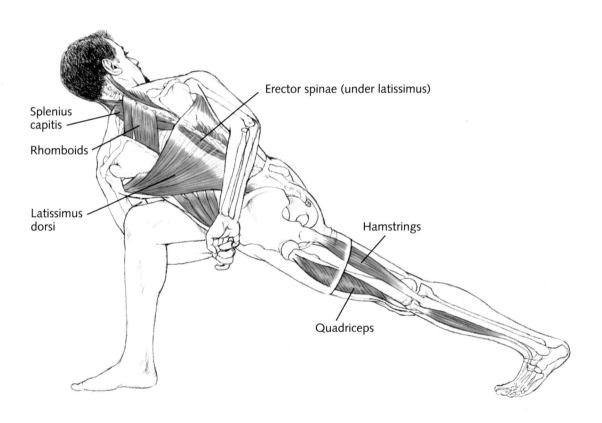

Erector spinae (under latissimus)

Splenius capitis

Rhomboids

Latissimus dorsi

Hamstrings

Quadriceps

Classification and Level

Advanced rotated asymmetrical standing pose

Joint Actions

Spinal axial rotation; scapula downward (medial) rotation; adduction right arm (abduction initially, then adduction in left arm as well); glenohumeral joints internal rotation, extension, adduction; elbow extension. Front leg: nutation, hip flexion and adduction, knee flexion, ankle dorsiflexion. Back leg: hip extension and adduction, knee extension.

The spinal rotation works the erector spinae and internal obliques on the side of the torso closer to the ceiling and the transversospinalis and rotatores and external obliques on the side of the torso closer to the front leg. All spinal extensors are active to counter the spinal flexion created by the action of the arms.

The arm binding works the supraspinatus to hold the head of the humerus in the socket, subscapularis, teres major, latissimus dorsi, and rhomboids, while lengthening the upper trapezius, pectoralis major, pectoralis minor, serratus anterior, supraspinatus, infraspinatus, teres minor, anterior deltoid, and coracobrachialis.

This arm binding also tends to create spinal flexion, combined with rotation, which is very challenging to the joints and discs in the spine. The force created by revolved side angle makes this a very powerful twist; it is possible to use the leverage of the arms in their binding and against the leg to force the spine past an appropriate range of motion. Because the lumbar spine is mostly incapable of axial rotation, overtwisting will stress the joints above and below: the sacroiliacs and T11-T12.

Obstacles and Notes

The anterior inferior part of the glenohumeral joint capsule is the most vulnerable to dislocation. The binding of the arms in internal rotation and extension puts pressure on this part of the joint capsule, especially if the scapulae are limited in their mobility. This caution applies to binding in general because it allows for more leverage or force to be directed into the joint.

Breathing

This pose is similar to revolved triangle, but more difficult because the strength, balance, and flexibility requirements are higher. The more open the pelvic structures are, the easier the balance and breathing will be. Here, the upper body is firmly bound in rotation against the resistance of the lower body, so there is significant resistance to the movements of the diaphragm, abdomen, and rib cage.

Trikonasana

Triangle Pose

trik-cone-AHS-anna

tri = three

kona = angle

Classification and Level

Basic hip-opening standing pose

Joint Actions

Spine neutral extension, slight rotation (but not much lateral extension); head axial rotation; upper limbs abduction, external rotation. Front leg: hip external rotation, flexion, abduction; knee extension; slight ankle plantarflexion; slight foot pronation. Back leg: hip internal rotation, adduction, extension; knee extension; foot supination.

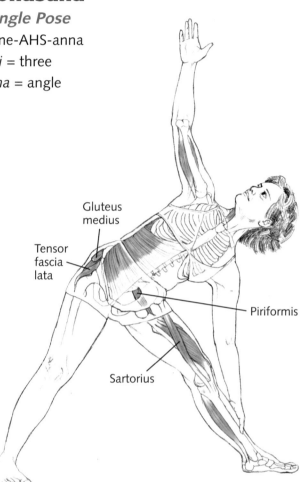

Gluteus medius

Tensor fascia lata

Piriformis

Sartorius

Working

Front leg: Iliacus, psoas major, piriformis, obturator internus (also as abductors), quadratus femoris, obturator externus, gemelli, gluteus medius and minimus, gluteus maximus (external rotation and abduction fibers), sartorius, hamstrings.

Back leg: Anterior fibers of gluteus medius and minimus, adductor magnus, gluteus maximus, pectineus, tensor fascia lata, semitendinosus, semimembranosus, biceps femoris.

Lengthening

Front leg: Quadratus femoris and obturator externus (working eccentrically as adductors), gemelli, pectineus, gracilis, adductor magnus and minimus, adductor longus and brevis, semitendinosus, semimembranosus, biceps femoris.

Back leg: Gluteus medius and minimus (eccentrically), gluteus maximus, sartorius, biceps femoris (eccentrically).

Obstacles and Notes

Pain or sensation in the medial knee of the front leg can be from the gracilis and semitendinosus, which are especially lengthened in this position and can transfer strain to the joint capsule.

It is important to keep the back of the front leg active (hamstrings) to avoid knee hyperextension, which is easy to do with the weight of the body over the leg. Sensations from within the knee (or any joint) are important signals to stop what you're doing and adjust your action or position.

Pain in the lateral knee of the back leg can be from tightness in the muscles at the top of the iliotibial band (tensor fascia lata, gluteus medius, gluteus maximus); they need to both lengthen and engage. If the gluteus medius and maximus are tight and the leg can't adduct relative to the pelvis, the spine will flex laterally. Tightness at the top of the iliotibial band can also contribute to tightness in the back of the ankle.

Does the spine rotate? The more articulate the sacroiliac joints, pelvic halves, and hip joints are, the more purely the spine can stay neutral. For example, if the front leg has a tight pectineus, the pelvis may rotate to the floor, and the spine will have to counterrotate more to open the chest. Restrictions in any of the other lower-body structures that need to articulate will produce similar compensatory changes farther up in the system.

Variation

Utthita Trikonasana

oo-TEE-tah trik-cone-AHS-anna

Extended Triangle Pose

utthita = extended

The extended version of triangle produces more acute angles between the legs and torso and the floor. All the same muscular actions apply, but at a greater range of motion. Even though extended triangle has a lower center of gravity, it is less stable than regular triangle, because the more extended this base of support becomes, the less able the supporting muscles will be to counter the downward pull of gravity on the pelvis and torso. If the pose becomes too extended, significant strain can be transferred to the joints and connective tissue of the weight-bearing structures.

Tensor fascia lata

Semitendinosus

Gracilis

Parivrtta Trikonasana

Revolved Triangle Pose

par-ee-vrit-tah trik-cone-AHS-anna

parivrtta = to turn around, revolve

tri = three

kona = angle

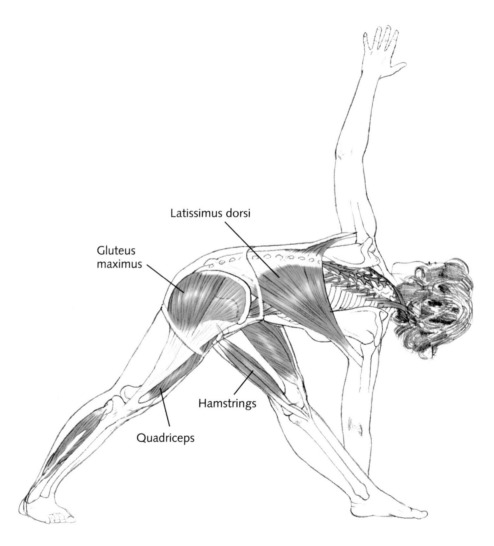

Classification and Level

Intermediate twisting asymmetrical standing pose

Joint Actions

Spine: Neutral extension, axial rotation.

Upper limbs: Abduction, external rotation, elbow extension.

Front leg: Hip flexion, adduction, external rotation; knee extension; ankle slight plantarflexion.

Back leg: Hip mild flexion, internal rotation; knee extension; ankle dorsiflexion; foot supinated at heel, pronated at forefoot.

Working

Transversospinalis group (especially multifidi), erector spinae group, internal and external obliques—to maintain neutral extension in the spine against the pull of gravity and the muscular efforts of the leg and pelvis.

Using Rotators and Abductors for Balance

Working while lengthening: Gluteus medius and minimus, quadratus femoris, obturator internus and externus, gemelli, piriformis.

Lengthening and releasing: Gluteus maximus, hamstrings, latissimus dorsi, teres major.

Obstacles and Notes

Weakness in the abductors and rotators will make eccentric control difficult. If this is the case, the gluteus maximus might be recruited, which will cause the pelvis to tilt posteriorly. The lower spine will then not be in neutral, and the rotation of the spine will not be around the head–tail axis.

Breathing

In revolved triangle, the more open the pelvic structures are, the easier the balance and breathing will be. Otherwise, the upper body will be held stiffly in rotation against the resistance of the lower body, and the diaphragm, abdomen, and rib cage will encounter considerable resistance to their movements.

Parsvottanasana

Intense Side Stretch

parsh-voh-tahn-AHS-anna

parsva = side, flank

ut = intense

tan = to stretch

Pelvic floor muscles

Gluteus medius

Erector spinae

Hamstrings

Gastrocnemius

Quadriceps

Soleus

Classification and Level

Basic asymmetrical forward-bending standing pose

Joint Actions

Spine flexion (mild); nutation in front leg; counternutation in back leg. Front leg: deep hip flexion, knee extension, ankle dorsiflexion. Back leg: hip flexion, medial rotation; knee extension; deep dorsiflexion in ankle.

Key Structures

Articulate pelvis and pelvic floor, hamstrings, feet and abductors for balance.

Working

Pelvic floor (to articulate sitting bones), quadriceps and articularis genus, abductors (gluteus medius and minimus for balance), feet and lower leg muscles (for balance).

Lengthening

Hamstrings (especially front leg), gluteus maximus (especially front leg), soleus and gastrocnemius (back leg), abductors, spinal erector muscles.

Obstacles

Tight hamstrings, gluteus maximus, soleus, gastrocnemius.

Weak or tight abductors will make it difficult to narrow stance.

Tight spinal muscles.

Notes

This forward bend is more intense in the hamstrings than uttanasana because the position of the back leg directs more of the flexion into the hip joint, and spinal flexibility is less of an issue.

Although the back leg is positioned with the leg turned out, the action of the muscles is toward internal rotation, to bring the pelvis into alignment (but not too much; can be overdone). The back foot also moves toward supination, to counter the inner rolling of the arch of the foot.

Breathing

The action of exhaling from the lower abdomen helps to position the pelvis on the thighs, and the action of inhaling into the thoracic region helps to lengthen the spine.

(continued)

Parsvottanasana Variation

With Arms in Reverse Namaskar

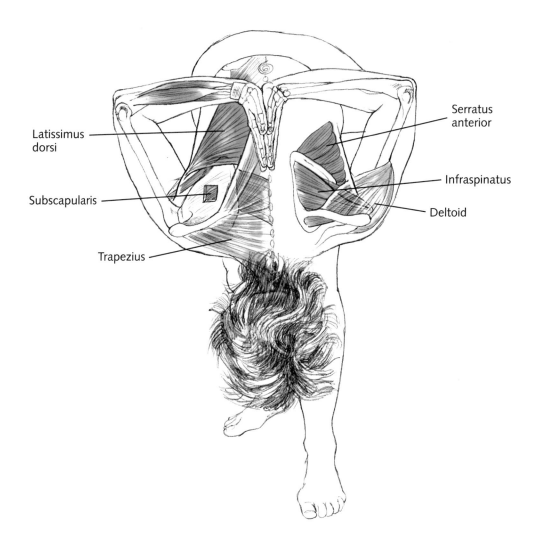

Latissimus dorsi

Subscapularis

Trapezius

Serratus anterior

Infraspinatus

Deltoid

Classification and Level

Intermediate asymmetrical forward-bending standing pose

Joint Actions

Downward rotation, adduction of scapulae on rib cage; extension and medial rotation at glenohumeral joint; elbow flexion; forearm pronation; wrist dorsiflexion; hand extension.

Key Structures

Scapulae articulating on rib cage, forearm and wrist mobility.

Working

Subscapularis; teres major; latissimus dorsi; rhomboids; lower, mid-, and upper trapezius.

Lengthening

Infraspinatus; teres minor; serratus anterior; anterior deltoids; pectoralis major and minor, if scapulae are adducted.

Obstacles

Overuse of the latissimus dorsi will interfere with the ability of the spine to flex.

Tight pectorals, tight deltoids, tight shoulder joint capsule.

Notes

This arm position is most easily done with the scapulae abducted. As the pose deepens, the scapulae move back into adduction.

Prasarita Padottanasana

Wide-Stance Forward Bend

pra-sa-REE-tah pah-doh-tahn-AHS-anna

prasarita = spread, expanded

pada = foot

ut = intense

tan = to stretch out

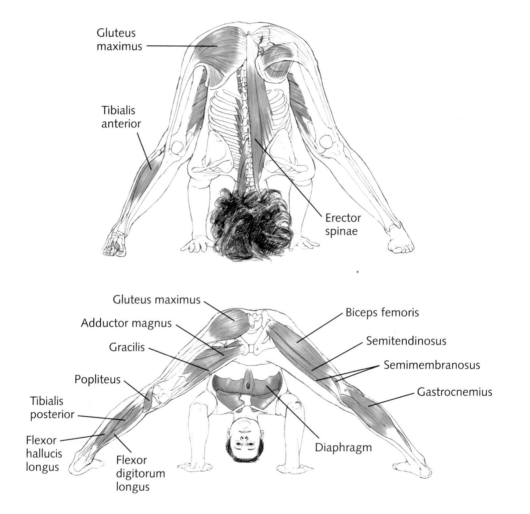

Classification and Level

Basic standing pose, inverted symmetrical forward bend

Joint Actions

Flexion and abduction at hips, knee extension, mild spinal flexion, mild medial rotation at hips or knees, pronation and supination at feet for balance.

Key Structures

Abductors and adductors of hips, medial hamstrings, ankles (feet and forelegs).

Working

Quadriceps and articularis genus (concentrically to bring knees into extension and keep kneecaps lifted); adductors (eccentrically, working against the body weight falling toward the floor); abductors (concentrically, to undo the knees falling inward and arches dropping); intrinsic and extrinsic muscles of the feet (to direct the weight through the calcaneus and not only the outer edge of the foot; the balance of supination and pronation is similar to the back leg in asymmetrical standing poses).

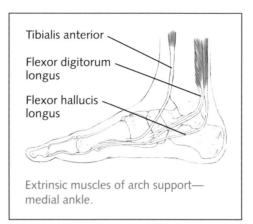

Tibialis anterior

Flexor digitorum longus

Flexor hallucis longus

Extrinsic muscles of arch support—medial ankle.

Lengthening

Adductors, in descending order: adductor magnus, adductor minimus, adductor longus, adductor brevis, gracilis—excepting pectineus (because of hip flexion, on slack). Hamstrings (particularly semitendinosus—the abduction of the legs puts more stretch into the medial hamstrings); spinal extensors; gluteus maximus, as part of hip flexion. If legs are medially rotated, may get some stretch through quadratus femoris, obturator externus.

As the legs separate (abduct), different hamstrings are affected more or less strongly as well as different adductors. Because some of the adductors also act as hip flexors, they aren't stretched in this position. The standing preparation for this pose (standing upright with the hips in neutral extension) would be more of a stretch for the pectineus and some fibers of the adductor brevis and gracilis.

Breathing

Wide-stance forward bend is probably the safest, most accessible inversion in all of yoga practice. The more firmly the legs can create support, while at the same time allowing the pelvis to freely rotate forward at the hip joints, the more relaxed the torso and breathing will be. This inversion provides mild traction and release to the spine, while reversing the usual action of the breath.

Hanging upside down, the diaphragm is pulled cranially by gravity, thus favoring the exhalation and the venous return from the lower body. While inhaling, the diaphragm pushes the weight of the abdominal organs caudally, against gravity, while at the same time mobilizing the costovertebral joints in the thoracic spine, which is being tractioned open. All these altered muscular actions can help normalize circulation in both muscles and organs that are constantly subjected to the usual stresses of upright weight bearing.

Upavesasana

Squat—Sitting-Down Pose

oo-pah-ve-SHAHS-anna

upavesa = sitting down, seat

Note: This pose is almost never referred to by a Sanskrit name, but there is some precedent for the name given here.

Classification and Level

Basic symmetrical standing pose

Joint Actions

Spinal axial extension; glenohumeral joint external rotation, adduction; elbow flexion; forearm pronation; wrist dorsiflexion; sacrum nutation; hip flexion, external rotation, abduction; knee flexion; ankle dorsiflexion.

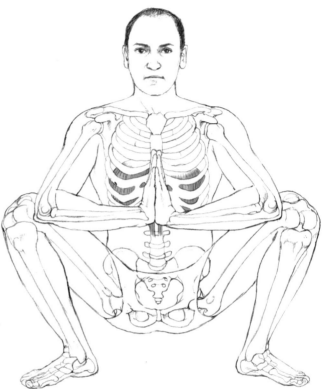

The pelvic floor can be contacted easily in this position, where it works synergistically to initiate exhaling, and releases some tone in response to the downward pressure exerted by the thoracic diaphragm when inhaling.

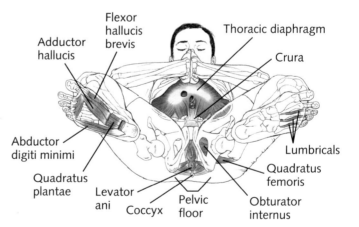

Note continuity of anterior longitudinal ligament with crura and coccyx.

Working

Pelvic floor: Obturator internus, levator ani. Isometrically: piriformis, obturator externus, two gemelli, quadratus femoris, biceps femoris, semitendinosus, semimembranosus, adductor magnus (long head). The legs should stay active; otherwise the deep flexion tends to collapse the hip joints, making it more challenging to activate the pelvic floor.

Foot: Lumbricals, quadratus plantae, adductor hallucis, flexor hallucis brevis, flexor digitorum brevis, opponens and flexor digiti minimi, abductor digiti minimi.

Lengthening

Adductor longus, adductor brevis, hamstrings, gastrocnemius, soleus, plantaris (not the gracilis, because of knee flexion).

Obstacles and Notes

The inability to dorsiflex the ankle deeply enough to keep the heels on the floor can be due to shortness in the Achilles tendon (specifically the soleus, in this position); however, restriction can also be in the front of the ankle. A quick fix is available by using support under the heels, but it's important not to become too reliant on it, because it will prevent activation of the intrinsic muscles of the feet, which stabilizes the arches, allows deeper flexion in the ankle, and aligns the bones of the foot and knee joint. Look for the tendon of the anterior tibialis popping forward; this is a telltale sign that deep support is lacking. Let gravity create the flexion, and use the intrinsic muscles to maintain integrity.

Breathing

This pose offers an opportunity to powerfully lengthen all three curves of the spine (axial extension). By definition this usually engages all three bandhas, and in this position, the deep support in the arches of the feet energetically feeds into the lifting action of the pelvic floor and lower abdominal muscles (mula bandha). The bracing of the elbows against the knees allows for a strong lengthening of the thoracic spine and lifting of the base of the rib cage and respiratory diaphragm (uddiyana bandha). The chin-lock of jalandhara bandha completes the action of axial extension and essentially freezes out the normal respiratory shape changes of breathing. This is when the unusual pattern of breath associated with mahamudra can arise deep in the core of the system (susumna).

SITTING POSES

CHAPTER **5**

For many people in the industrialized world, sitting (or more likely, slouching) on a piece of furniture is the body position in which they spend most of their waking hours. What shoes are to the feet, chairs, car seats, and couches are to the pelvic joints and lower spine.

In India, even well-to-do families frequently eschew the use of furniture in their homes—preferring to sit, dine, and sometimes even sleep on the floor. Not surprisingly, the Western epidemic of lower-back pain is almost unknown in that part of the world.

In yoga practice, just as the bare feet develop a new relationship with the ground through the practice of standing asanas, the hip, pelvic joints, and lower spine develop a new relationship with the earth when you bear weight directly on them in sitting postures.

The asanas depicted in this chapter are either sitting positions themselves or are entered into from sitting. If practiced with attention to the anatomy of the relevant joints, muscles, and connective tissue, they can help to restore some of the natural flexibility you knew as a child, when sitting and playing on the floor for hours at a time was effortless.

Beyond the idea of restoring natural function to the pelvis and lower back, yogic sitting also has an association with more advanced practices. The word *asana* in fact can be literally translated as "seat," and from a certain perspective, all of asana practice can be viewed as a methodical way of freeing up the spine, limbs, and breathing so that the yogi can spend extended periods of time in a seated position. In this most stable of body shapes, the distractions of dealing with gravity and breath can disappear, freeing the body's energies for the deeper contemplative work of meditative practices.

Sukhasana

Easy Posture

suk-HAS-anna

sukha = comfortable, gentle, agreeable

Beginning seated pose

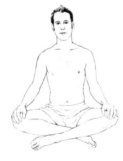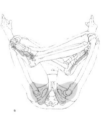

Siddhasana

Adept's Posture

sid-DHAS-anna

siddha = accomplished, fulfilled, perfected

Basic seated pose

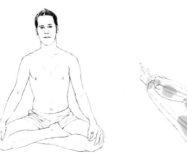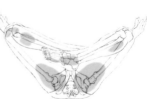

Blue shaded areas indicate places of contact with the floor.

Svastikasana

Auspicious Posture

sva-steek-AHS-anna

svastik = lucky or auspicious

Intermediate seated pose

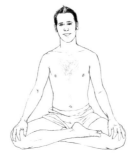
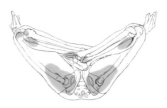

Padmasana

Lotus Posture

pod-MAHS-anna

padma = lotus

Advanced seated pose

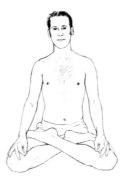
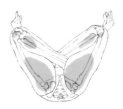

Mulabandhasana

Pose of the Root Lock

moola-ban-DHAS-anna

mula = root, foundation, bottom

bandha = binding, tying, a bond

Very advanced seated axial extension

Pose used for pranayama

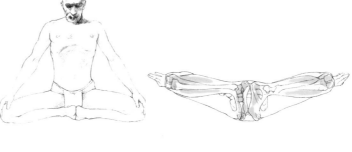

Key structures for all seated poses

Feet, ankles, knees, hip joints, pelvis, spine, and skull.

Common joint actions

Knees flexed

Hip joints flexed

Spine in neutral curves or axial extension

Skull balanced on spine

Common elements to all sitting

Whatever sitting position one chooses, if the knees are above the hip joints, the pelvis can tip posteriorly, causing the spinal curves to go into flexion, especially if there is tightness in the hamstrings. To maintain an upright shape, the erector muscles contract to extend the spine, and the psoas muscles contract to pull the anterior lumbar spine forward (attempting to restore the lumbar curve). Unfortunately, this psoas action tends to also pull the hips into greater flexion, reinforcing the posterior tilt of the pelvis, which calls a host of other muscles into play in attempt to compensate. A person engaged in such a losing battle with gravity will have little energy available for breathing or meditation practices, and will soon tire of sitting.

In order for a seated asana to be maintained in a comfortable manner for any length of time, for most people, the hip joints need to be at least slightly elevated above the knees. For the vast majority of people, this requires the use of a cushion, folded blanket, or other aid.[1] With the hips elevated above the knees, the lumbar and other spinal curves are restored, and the weight of the head can balance with minimal muscular effort. In a well-supported seated asana, the intrinsic equilibrium of the pelvis, spine, and breathing mechanism support the body, and the energy that has been liberated from postural effort can be focused on deeper processes, such as breathing or meditation.

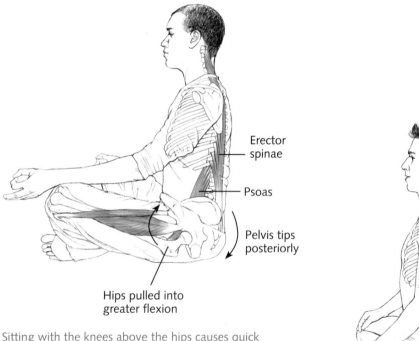

Erector
spinae

Psoas

Pelvis tips
posteriorly

Hips pulled into
greater flexion

Sitting with the knees above the hips causes quick
fatigue because the muscles must work against gravity.

Spinal
curves
restored

Sitting with the hips above the knees
restores equilibrium and allows for
longer comfort.

[1] The less flexible the individual, the higher the support must be. For some, no amount of support will create a comfortable seat on the floor; that is an indication that a chair should be used for seated practices.

Paschimottanasana

West (Back) Stretching

POS-chee-moh-tan-AHS-anna

pascha = behind, after, later, westward

uttana = intense stretch

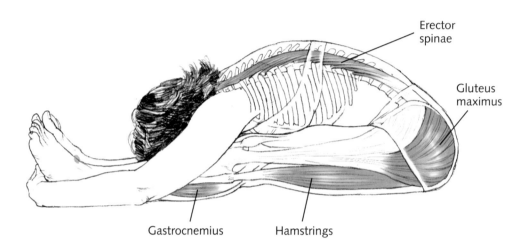

Erector spinae

Gluteus maximus

Gastrocnemius   Hamstrings

The back of the body is referred to as "west" due to the traditional practice of facing the rising sun when performing morning worship. Compare with purvotta-nasana—a stretch for the front of the body (*purva* = in front, before, eastward).

Classification and Level

Basic seated forward bend

Joint Actions

Spinal flexion (moving toward extension); sacrum nutation; hip flexion, adduction, internal rotation; knee extension; ankle slight dorsiflexion; scapula abduction, upward rotation; glenohumeral joint flexion, slight external rotation, adduction; elbow extension; forearm slight pronation.

Working

Gravity acts to pull the torso toward the top of the thighs.

Spine: Extensors can act to deepen action in the hip joints.

Legs: Vastii and articularis genus to extend knees.

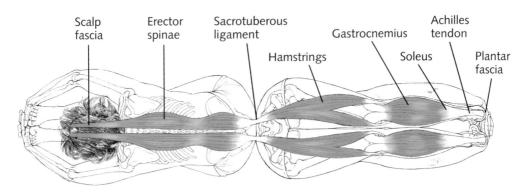

Scalp fascia   Erector spinae   Sacrotuberous ligament   Gastrocnemius   Achilles tendon

Hamstrings   Soleus   Plantar fascia

The back line of the body is a continuous network of muscle and fascia that extends from the soles of the feet (plantar fascia) to the scalp fascia and the ridge of the brow.

Lengthening

Spine: Spinal extensors (if releasing into pose), latissimus dorsi.

Legs: Hamstrings, gluteus maximus, piriformis, obturator internus and gemelli, gluteus medius and minimus, gastrocnemius and soleus; popliteus works at length (eccentrically) to prevent hyperextension of the knees.

Arms: Rhomboids, lower trapezius, latissimus dorsi.

Obstacles and Notes

If there is a lot of tightness in the hamstrings and gluteus maximus, hip flexion will be restricted and the hip flexors (psoas major, iliacus, pectineus, and rectus femoris) and abdominal muscles will tend to contract to pull the body forward into this pose. Instead, a folded blanket under the sitting bones can elevate the seat so that gravity is drawing the upper body forward more effectively. This is preferable to using the hip flexors and abdominal muscles, which can create a sense of congestion in the hip joints.

Elevating the seat, bending the knees, or both, can allow the spine to come more forward. There will still be lengthening in the hamstrings, but in a less stressful way.

It should be noted that any stretching sensations around the origin or insertion of a muscle indicate that the tendons and connective tissue are being stretched— as opposed to the muscle fibers. Alignment and intention should always be adapted to direct stretching sensations into the belly of the target muscle—not its attachments.

Breathing

The breath can be very helpful while moving into this pose. Emphasizing the action of the exhalation deepens the flexion at the pelvis, whereas emphasizing the action of the inhalation assists in extending the upper spine. This will only occur if the exhalation is initiated with the lower abdominal muscles and the inhalation is directed toward the rib cage.

Janu Sirsasana

Head-to-Knee Pose

JAH-new shear-SHAHS-anna

janu = knee

shiras = to touch with the head

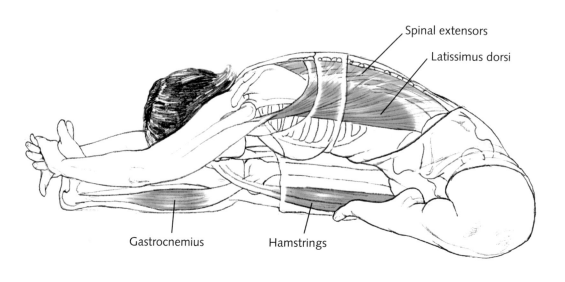

Spinal extensors

Latissimus dorsi

Gastrocnemius

Hamstrings

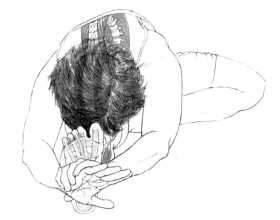

The entire back line of the extended leg side can be lengthened—from the sole of the foot to the scalp fascia.

Classification and Level

Intermediate seated forward bend

Joint Actions

Mild spinal flexion (moving toward extension) and mild rotation; sacrum is in nutation. Extended leg: hip flexion, adduction, internal rotation; knee extension; ankle is in dorsiflexion. Folded leg: hip flexion, abduction, external rotation; knee flexion; ankle plantarflexion; foot supination. Shoulders and arms: scapula abduction, upward rotation; glenohumeral joint flexion, slight external rotation, adduction; elbow extension; forearm slight pronation.

Working

Gravity acts to pull the torso toward the extended leg.

Spine: Spinal extensors can act to deepen the action in the hip joints. Extended-leg-side internal obliques and folded-leg-side external obliques act together to rotate the spine to face the extended leg. The folded-leg-side rotatores and multifidi act to rotate the spine toward the extended leg.

Extended leg: Gravity acts to flex the hip; the vastii and articularis genus extend the knees (if necessary).

Folded leg: Gravity acts to nutate the sacrum and flex the hip. The obturator externus, quadratus femoris, piriformis, obturator internus, and gemelli externally rotate the hip; the sartorius externally rotates and flexes the hip and knee. The hamstrings act to flex the knee, and the tibialis anterior flexes the ankle and supinates the foot.

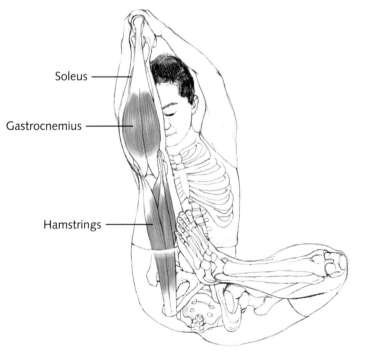

Soleus

Gastrocnemius

Hamstrings

Janu sirsasana from underneath.

(continued)

Lengthening

Spine: The spinal extensors lengthen if releasing into the pose. The latissimus dorsi lengthen bilaterally. Extended-leg-side external obliques and folded-leg-side internal obliques, extended-leg-side rotatores, and multifidi lengthen with the rotation toward the straight leg (these are the reverse of the working actions mentioned earlier).

Extended leg: Hamstrings, gluteus maximus, piriformis, obturator internus and gemelli, some gluteus medius and minimus, gastrocnemius, and soleus. The popliteus can create slight knee flexion to prevent hyperextension.

Folded leg: The adductor magnus mainly stretches because it creates internal rotation, extension, and adduction (as in baddha konasana). The adductor longus and brevis also stretch because they flex and externally rotate the leg (abduction lengthens these two). The more the legs are externally rotated and abducted, the more the pectineus is lengthened. There also might be some lengthening in the tensor fascia lata, because of the external rotation, and in the fibers of the gluteus medius and minimus with increasing hip flexion.

Arms: The rhomboids lengthen, as do the lower trapezius and latissimus dorsi.

Obstacles and Notes

The asymmetry of this pose makes it very revealing about the "sidedness" exhibited in the back muscles. Janu sirsasana can also reveal sidedness in the relative stability or mobility of the sacroiliac joints. Everyone has an "easy" and a "hard" side in this pose because of the inherent asymmetries of the human body.

The more mobile the sacroiliac joint is on the side of the flexed leg, the easier it is to turn and face the extended leg. This is especially true as the spine extends toward the extended leg. As hip flexion deepens, less spinal flexion is required. Because this limits even further the rotation in the lumbar spine, more movement needs to happen at the sacroiliac joint.

It is very common to overmobilize the sacroiliac joint in janu sirsasana. This happens when the pose is pushed or flexed too forcibly or held for too long without relieving the weight on the pelvis. Alternatively, immobility of the pelvic joints can lead to excessive torque in the bent-leg knee joint. Many yogis report meniscus tears occurring as they move into this pose. This happens in a partially flexed knee as the pelvis flexes forward, taking the femur with it, which grinds the medial femoral condyle into the medial meniscus. Ensuring that the bent leg is truly fully flexed will move the meniscus safely to the back of the joint.

All this points to the fact that the potential stresses to the spine, sacroiliac, and hip and knee joints need to be evenly distributed so that no one structure takes all the force of this pose.

Breathing

The breath can be very helpful while moving into this pose. Emphasizing the action of the exhalation deepens the flexion at the pelvis, whereas emphasizing the action of the inhalation assists in extending the upper spine. This will only occur if the exhalation is initiated with the lower abdominal muscles and the inhalation is directed toward the rib cage.

It's interesting to experiment with the opposite pattern of breath, just to create a contrast: Try exhaling by compressing the chest and inhaling into the belly region. Notice the effect on the asana compared with the first suggestions.

Parivrtta Janu Sirsasana

Revolved Head-to-Knee Pose

par-ee-vrit-tah JAH-new shear-SHAHS-anna

parivrtta = turning, rolling

janu = knee

shiras = to touch with the head

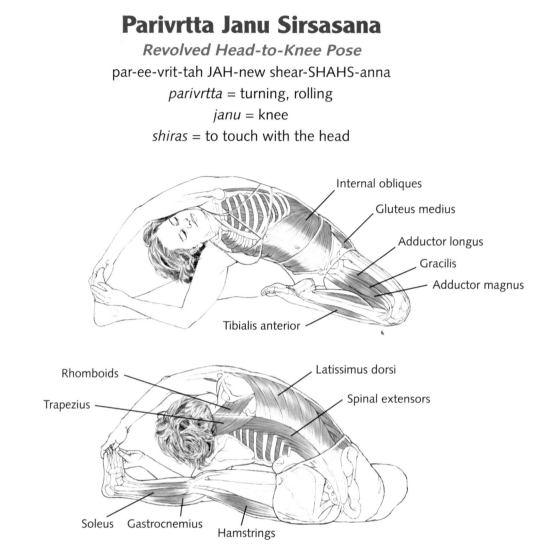

Classification and Level

Intermediate seated lateral twist

Joint Actions

Spinal rotation and lateral flexion. Extended leg: hip flexion, adduction, internal rotation; knee extension; ankle slight dorsiflexion. Folded leg: hip flexion, abduction, external rotation; knee flexion; ankle plantarflexion; foot supination. Shoulders and arms: scapula upward rotation, elevation, adduction; glenohumeral joint flexion, external rotation; elbow extension; forearm supination.

Working

Gravity pulls the torso into lateral flexion.

Spine: Bent-leg-side internal obliques and extended-leg-side external obliques to rotate the spine away from the extended leg; extended-leg-side rotatores and multifidi to rotate the spine toward the folded leg.

Extended leg: Gravity to flex the hip; vastii and articularis genus to extend the knees (if necessary).

Flexed leg: Obturator externus and quadratus femoris, piriformis, obturator internus and gemelli to externally rotate; sartorius to externally rotate and flex the hip and knee; hamstrings to flex the knee; tibialis anterior to supinate the foot.

Lengthening

Spine: Spinal extensors, quadratus lumborum, and latissimus dorsi on top side; top side external obliques; lower side rotatores and multifidi lengthen with rotation toward the folded leg.

Extended leg: Hamstrings, gluteus maximus, piriformis, obturator internus and gemelli, gluteus medius and minimus, gastrocnemius, soleus, popliteus.

Folded leg: Adductor magnus mainly (because it creates internal rotation, extension, and adduction), adductor longus and brevis (because they flex and externally rotate the leg; abduction lengthens these two), some pectineus (the more the legs are externally rotated and abducted, the more the pectineus is lengthened). There also might be some lengthening in the tensor fascia lata with the external rotation and in the fibers of the gluteus medius and minimus with more flexion.

Arms: Rhomboids, lower trapezius, latissimus dorsi.

Obstacles and Notes

Although the legs in this pose are the same as in janu sirsasana, the action in the spine is very different: Instead of rotating toward the extended leg, the rotation is away from the leg, and instead of flexion in the spine there is lateral flexion. This change in spinal action changes the action in the shoulder girdle and arms as well—notably, more lengthening occurs in the latissimus dorsi.

Side-bending poses are great for releasing restrictions in the shoulder joints. When flexion of the glenohumeral joint is restricted, greater mobility can often be found by mobilizing the scapula in lateral flexion.

In this pose, the opposite sitting bone must stay on the ground to keep the pose's action balanced. When side bending over the extended leg, the hip of the folded leg can come off the floor, which diminishes the lengthening in the back of the body, but increases the lengthening in the back of the extended leg.

Breathing

The upper side of this pose is receiving more stretch, and the rib cage is more open, but the lower dome of the diaphragm is more mobile, and the lower lung's tissue is more compliant. Focusing on this fact can quite naturally create a bit more awareness of the lower side, which helps prevent compressive collapse.

Upavistha Konasana

Seated Wide-Angle Pose

oo-pah-VEESH-tah cone-AHS-anna

upavistha = seated

kona = angle

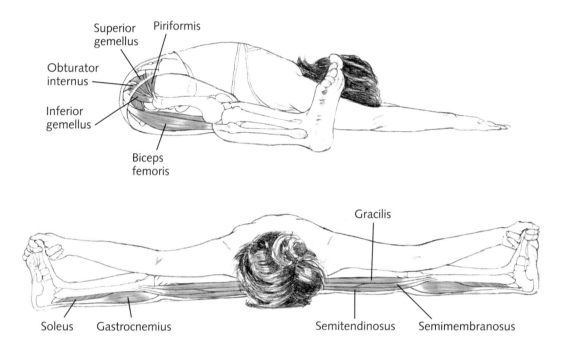

Classification and Level

Intermediate seated forward bend

Joint Actions

Mild spinal flexion (moving toward axial extension); sacrum nutation; major hip abduction, external rotation, and flexion; knee extension; ankle dorsiflexion.

Working

Legs: The gemelli and obturator internus are doing both external rotation and abduction. To a lesser degree, the piriformis and gluteus maximus can help with external rotation (but are also hip extensors); additionally, the obturator externus and quadratus femoris can help with external rotation (but are also adductors). The posterior fibers of the gluteus medius and minimus help somewhat with abduction, but are working at a pretty short length, so they may cramp.

Spine: Spinal extensors are active here so that as the pose deepens and the head comes forward to reach the floor, the spine flattens out along the floor. If too much emphasis is put on flexing the spine to get the head down, the legs are not adequately accessed.

Lengthening

Legs: Piriformis and gluteus maximus are working eccentrically because they are extensors of the hip; obturator externus and quadratus femoris are working eccentrically because they are also adductors. Of the adductors, the gracilis is especially stretched because of the knee extension; the pectineus is not affected because of the hip flexion. In the hamstrings, the semi-tendinosus and semimembranosus are particularly lengthened here because of the abduction of the legs. When the hands reach to the foot to assist the ankle into dorsiflexion, the gastrocnemius receives a strong stretch.

Piriformis

Gemellus

Obturator internus

Gracilis

Spine: Extensors of the spine are lengthening, but active. As the pose deepens, it moves toward more axial extension.

Obstacles and Notes

There is a strong action of nutation at the sacroiliac joint, as the top of the sacrum "nods" forward, while leaving the iliac bones behind.

If the legs roll inward, there can be too much stretch for the inner knee and adductors. For tight students, it's preferable to bend the knees a bit (with support) so that the stretching sensations are felt more in the bellies of the relevant muscles. Sensations of stretch occurring near the joints and muscle attachments are indicators that nothing useful is likely to result from the stretch.

Breathing

The act of gradually lengthening the spine in this pose can be greatly assisted by the breath. The exhalation, if initiated in the lower abdomen, can help anchor the sitting bones and ground the backs of the thighs, whereas the inhalation, if it's initiated in the upper chest, can help to lengthen the spine. In short, the exhalation can ground the posture's lower half, and the inhalation can lengthen the posture's upper half.

Baddha Konasana

Bound Angle Pose

BAH-dah cone-AHS-anna

baddha = bound

kona = angle

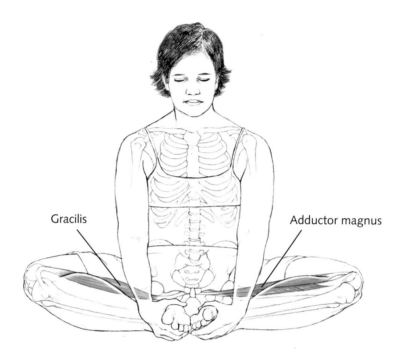

Gracilis

Adductor magnus

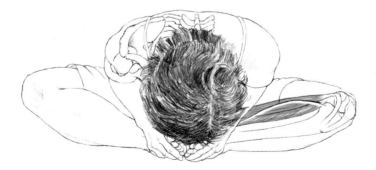

Classification and Level

Basic seated hip/groin stretch

Joint Actions

Spine neutral extension when upright, moving to mild flexion when bending forward (but not too much flexion, which will reduce the action in the pelvis); sacroiliac joint nutation; hip flexion and external rotation; knee flexion; ankle dorsiflexion; foot supination; scapula neutral on rib cage; glenohumeral joint external rotation, anatomically neutral; elbow flexion; forearm supination; hand and finger flexion.

Working

Spine: Intertransversarii, interspinalis, rotatores, transversospinalis group, erector spinae group to maintain neutral extension of spine, then gravity to bring the spine forward and into mild flexion.

Legs: Gravity nutates the sacrum and flexes the hips; the obturator externus, quadratus femoris, piriformis, obturator internus, and gemelli act to externally rotate the hip joint; the hamstrings work to flex the knees; the tibialis anterior supinates the foot. The sartorius should be considered active as well, to flex and externally rotate the hip joint.

Arms: A balance between the serratus anterior and rhomboids is needed to hold the scapulae on the rib cage. The biceps flex the elbows and draw the body forward, as the flexors of the carpals and fingers work to grasp the feet.

Lengthening

Legs: A major stretch is given to the adductor magnus mainly because it creates internal rotation, extension, and adduction, opposite to the actions of baddha konasana. There is also some stretch to the adductor longus and brevis, and gracilis. The more the knees are extended, the more the gracilis is lengthened. Because the adductor longus and brevis work to flex and externally rotate the leg, it's the abduction in the pose that lengthens these two of the adductor group.

There also might be some lengthening in the tensor fascia latae, as a result of external rotation, and in the fibers of the gluteus medius and minimus with increased hip flexion. The hamstrings will also lengthen with increased hip flexion, increasing as the feet move away and the knees extend more.

Obstacles and Notes

Much as in paschimottanasana, if the focus is too much on getting the head down, the resulting action is more spinal (flexion) than pelvic (sacroiliac and hip joints). For this reason, the intention should not be to get the head to the feet, but to get the navel to the feet.

(continued)

The activity of the obturator internus in this pose also activates the muscles of the pelvic floor. This is an opportunity to engage mula bandha, which anchors the base of the pose.

Depending on how close the feet are to the groin, different external rotators will be activated to assist with rotating the legs out and different adductors will be lengthened. Thus, it's quite valuable to work with the feet at different distances from the pelvis. Closer isn't always better.

Baddha konasana can be challenging for the knees. The supination of the feet (soles toward the ceiling) causes a rotation of the tibia that, combined with flexion, destabilizes the ligamentous support for the knees. If the hips are not very mobile and the legs are pushed into this pose, the lower leg torque can travel into the knee joints. One way to protect them is to evert the foot (press the outer edges into the floor). This activates the peroneals, which, via fascial connections, can stabilize the lateral ligaments of the knees and help to keep them from rotating too much. The result of this will be to direct more of the pose's action into the hip joints.

Breathing

The advice to bring the navel—rather than the head—to the feet is another way of saying that the breath should remain as unobstructed as possible in this pose. Pushing the head toward the floor will collapse the rib cage and compress the abdomen, resulting in a reduced ability for those cavities to change shape. A lengthened spine results in freer breathing.

Variation

Supta Baddha Konasana

Reclining Bound Angle Pose
   supta = resting, lain down to sleep

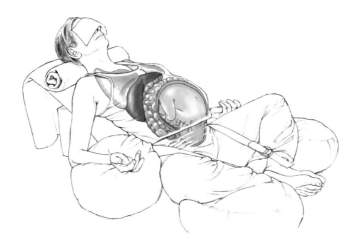

This restful variation of baddha konasana puts the spine in neutral alignment or very mild extension to gently open up the breathing. It is a very commonly used restorative posture, and by using props such as bolsters, blankets, straps, and cushions, it can be modified in a wide variety of ways.

Ardha Matsyendrasana

Half Lord of the Fishes Pose

ARD-hah MOTS-yen-DRAHS-anna

ardha = half

matsya = fish

indra = ruler, lord

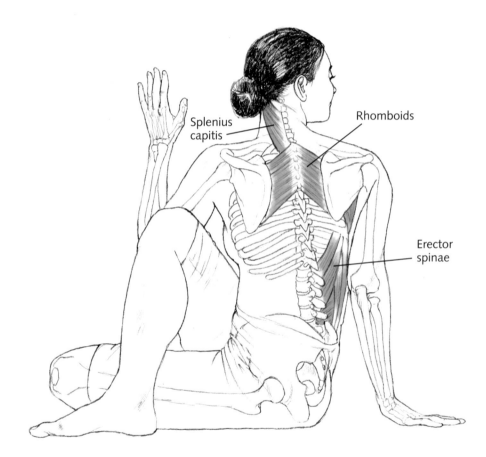

Sage Matsyenda was a renowned teacher of yoga who, according to legend, developed this pose.

Classification and Level

Basic seated twisting pose

There are a variety of more advanced bound arm positions, but we have chosen to analyze this simpler arm placement.

Actions

Spinal rotation toward raised (top) leg, neutral extension. Top leg: deep hip flexion, adduction, internal rotation; knee flexion. Bottom leg: moderate hip flexion, adduction, external rotation; knee flexion. Front arm (contralateral arm rests on top leg): scapula in neutral, glenohumeral external rotation, slight abduction, and flexion moving toward extension; elbow flexion; wrist neutral extension. Back arm: scapula neutral; glenohumeral external rotation, extension; elbow extension; wrist dorsiflexion.

Working

Spine: Top leg side: internal obliques, erector spinae, splenius capitis. Bottom leg side: external obliques, rotatores, and multifidi; sternocleidomastoid; spinal extensors to maintain extension and resist flexion of the spine against the pressure of the arm.

Legs: Top: adduction and internal rotation with gracilis, pectineus, adductor magnus. Bottom: hamstrings to flex knee, gravity.

Arms: Front: rhomboids to maintain the placement of the scapula on the rib cage against the resistance of the leg; infraspinatus and teres minor to externally rotate the humerus; posterior deltoid to laterally abduct the arm against the leg; biceps to flex the elbow. Back: infraspinatus and teres minor; serratus anterior to keep the scapula placed on the rib cage and resist adduction of this scapula.

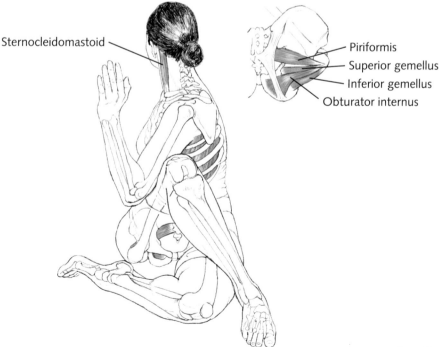

Sternocleidomastoid

Piriformis
Superior gemellus
Inferior gemellus
Obturator internus

(continued)

Lengthening

Spine: Bottom leg side: internal obliques, erector spinae, splenius capitis, latissimus dorsi. Top leg side: external obliques, rotatores, and multifidi; sternocleidomastoid.

Legs: Top: piriformis with internal hip rotation, adduction, and flexion; gemelli and obturator internus with internal rotation and adduction; quadratus femoris and obturator externus with internal rotation; gluteus maximus because of internal rotation and flexion; gluteus medius and minimus because of adduction. Bottom: piriformis because of hip adduction and flexion; gluteus medius and minimus because of hip adduction and flexion.

Arms: Front: rhomboids may be working eccentrically and lengthening; latissimus dorsi may be lengthening because of external shoulder rotation and rotation of the spine. Back: pectoralis major, long head of biceps, pectoralis minor, coracobrachialis.

Obstacles and Notes

All parts of the torso can contribute to this twist—both right and left sides of the front and both right and left sides of the back, at different layers of muscle. The spine will have the most balanced rotation when in neutral extension. Flexion in the lumbar spine will jeopardize the stability of the lumbar vertebrae and discs, and too much extension will tend to lock the thoracic spine into place, inhibiting axial rotation there.

The twisting action of this pose can be "faked" by overmobilizing the scapulae and allowing them to adduct (the back one) and abduct (the front one) excessively. When this happens there is the appearance of rotation, but not much actual movement in the spine. Because the shoulder girdle has more range of motion in this direction than the thoracic structures have, it is frequently a more intense spinal twist when the arms are placed in a simple, nonbound position. It is therefore preferable to enter this pose without using the arms, so the maximum safe action is found in the spine. The leverage of the arms comes in last, as a deepening, stabilizing (not mobilizing) action. Overuse of the arms can direct too much force into vulnerable parts of the spine—particularly T11-T12.

Another factor that contributes to the intensity of the spinal twisting action of this pose is the arrangement of the legs, which greatly limits rotational movements in the pelvis—and in fact counterrotates the pelvis away from the rotation of the spine.

Breathing

Ardha matsyendrasana provides a very clear opportunity to explore the basic dynamics of the breath as they relate to the principles of brahmana/langhana, prana/apana, and sthira/sukha.

The lower body is the stable base of the pose, and a langhana "belly breathing" pattern can release tension in the lower abdomen, hip joints, and pelvic floor. This approach to breathing stimulates the experience of apana flowing downward in the system, into the earth.

The upper body is the mobile, supported aspect of the pose, and the brahmana "chest breath" can be accomplished here simply by stabilizing the abdominal wall upon the initiation of the inhalation. This will drive the diaphragm's action into the rib cage and costovertebral articulations and greatly intensify deep rotational release in the thoracic spine. This breathing pattern is clearly related to the upward movement of apana, using the lower abdominal muscles to assist in driving the exhalation upward and outward from the body.

In this pose, use a simple nonbound arm position and try doing several rounds of relaxed belly breathing to begin with. Then, gradually deepen the lower abdominal contractions on the exhalation, eventually maintaining that contraction for a moment when initiating the next inhalation. Notice the effect of the breathing patterns on your experience of the pose.

Dandasana

Staff Pose

dan-DAHS-anna

danda = stick, staff

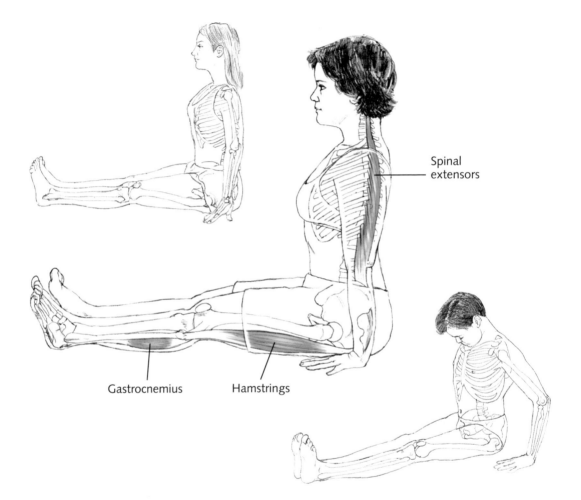

Arm and torso proportions: short, neutral, and long.

Classification and Level

Basic seated neutral extension

Joint Actions

Spine neutral or axial extension; sacroiliac is neutral; hip flexion to 90 degrees, adduction and internal rotation; knee extension; ankle dorsiflexion; scapula neutral on rib cage; glenohumeral neutral extension; elbow extension; wrist dorsiflexion (depending on arm length).

Working

Spine: All spinal extensors, the psoas major and minor.

Legs: The iliacus to flex the hips, the pectineus and adductor magnus to adduct and internally rotate the legs. The vastii extend the knees. (If this amount of flexion is challenging, the pectineus or rectus femoris might overwork to pull the pelvis into flexion against the backward pull of gravity.)

Arms: The serratus anterior resists the adduction of the scapulae resulting from the push of the arms; the triceps extend the elbows. The flexor carpi radialis and ulnaris, and the lumbricals of the hands, support the arch of the hand and prevent overflexing of the wrist (short-armed people would need a block under each hand to create this action).

Lengthening

Legs: The hamstrings, gluteus maximus, piriformis, obturator internus, and gemelli all lengthen. Additionally, there will be some lengthening in the gluteus medius and minimus, as well as the gastrocnemius and soleus. Working at length (eccentrically) is the popliteus.

Arms: Depending on arm length, the biceps may be lengthening.

Obstacles and Notes

This pose clearly reveals how tightness in the legs can create spinal flexion. Obstacles that show up clearly in this pose are often the cause of difficulties in more complex poses, where the restrictions are less obvious. For example, tightness in the legs will affect downward-facing dog, but in a way that can appear to be more about shoulder or spinal restriction.

Not everyone can use their arms to help create the neutral spinal extension in dandasana due to proportional differences in arm-to-body length. Conversely, what appears to be different arm-to-body proportions can sometimes be the result of chronically elevated or depressed positioning of the scapulae on the rib cage. Additionally, if the spine is unable to extend into vertical because of tightness in the hips and legs, the arms may seem too long.

For students of vinyasa flows that involve jump-throughs, knowing your arm-to-torso proportions is absolutely essential. An inability to jump-through due to a long torso and short arms will not respond to any amount of stretching or strengthening. Use blocks under the hands to level the playing field.

Breathing

This is a straight-legged opportunity to breathe into an axially extended spine (mahamudra). Unlike pada hastasana, in which the legs are working to support the weight of the body, the legs are not "naturally" activated in dandasana. For this reason, the work in the legs is quite different, and for most people, more difficult to maintain. All three bandhas can be employed here, but it's quite a challenge to do even 10 breaths while maintaining them with the proper body alignment.

Gomukhasana

Cow-Faced Pose

go-moo-KAHS-anna

go = cow

mukha = face

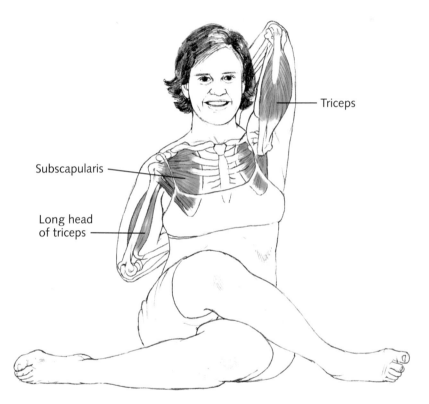

Triceps

Subscapularis

Long head
of triceps

Classification and Level

Intermediate hip and shoulder opener

Joint Actions

Mostly neutral spine, with slight extension in the thoracic spine because of the
arm position. Top arm: scapula upward rotation, elevation, adduction; glenohumeral joint external rotation and flexion; elbow flexion; forearm pronation. Bottom arm: scapula downward rotation, adduction, depression;
glenohumeral joint internal rotation, extension; elbow flexion; forearm
supination. Legs: hip flexion, external rotation, adduction; knee flexion;
ankle plantarflexion.

Working

Legs: Because this is a hip opener, the leg and hip muscles are released into gravity as much as possible.

Arms: Top arm: infraspinatus and teres minor for external rotation, serratus anterior to upwardly rotate scapula, then rhomboids to adduct, anterior deltoid to flex arm, pronator teres, finger flexors. Bottom arm: subscapularis to internally rotate, teres major and latissimus dorsi for internal rotation and extension, long head of triceps and posterior deltoids to extend arm, biceps to flex elbow, supinators in forearm, finger flexors.

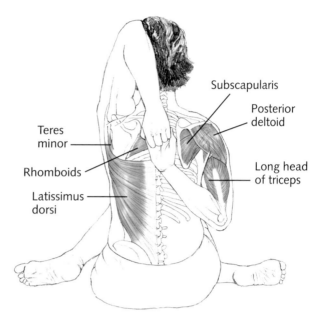

Subscapularis
Posterior deltoid
Teres minor
Rhomboids
Latissimus dorsi
Long head of triceps

Lengthening

Legs: Abductors (gluteus medius, minimus, maximus) and extensors (adductor magnus and hamstrings); piriformis because of flexion and adduction of legs.

Arms: Top arm: triceps, latissimus dorsi, teres major, pectoralis minor and pectoralis major. Bottom arm: long head of biceps, pectoralis major, serratus anterior, upper trapezius.

Obstacles and Notes

Upward and downward rotation of the scapula needs to precede adduction to avoid overmobilizing in the shoulder joint. If the scapulae don't mobilize, there can be too much movement in the glenohumeral joint causing overstretching in the joint capsule or impingements in the tendons of the biceps and supraspinatus.

If the hips joints are not sufficiently mobile, excessive torque can result in the knee joints. Great care should be taken to avoid any strain in the knees, because the menisci are most vulnerable when the knee joints are semiflexed.

Breathing

Releasing the abdominal wall and directing the breath into the lower abdomen helps the pelvic floor and hip joints to release. Restraining the lower abdomen during an inhalation directs the breath into the thoracic region, which intensifies the stretching in the shoulder structures.

Hanumanasana

Monkey Pose

ha-new-mahn-AHS-anna

hanumat = having large jaws: a monkey-chief

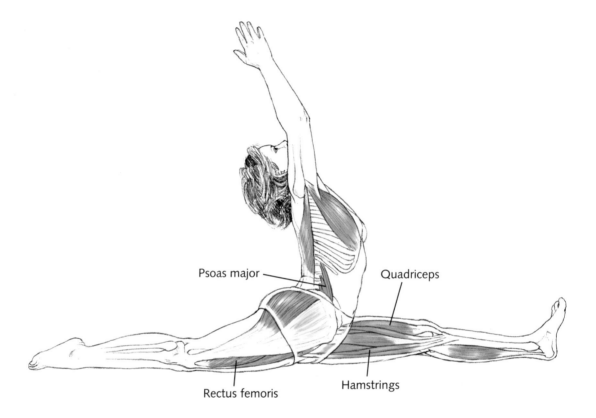

Psoas major

Quadriceps

Rectus femoris

Hamstrings

Hanuman was the semidivine chief of an army of monkeys who served the god Rama. As told in the Hindu epic, the Ramayana, Hanuman once jumped in a single stride the distance between Southern India and (Sri) Lanka. This split-leg pose mimics his famous leap.

Classification and Level

Advanced seated split

Joint Actions

Spinal extension. Front leg: sacrum nutation; hip flexion, internal rotation, adduction; knee extension; ankle neutral extension. Back leg: sacrum counternutation; hip extension, internal rotation, adduction; knee extension; ankle plantarflexion; scapula upward rotation, abduction, elevation; glenohumeral joint flexion, adduction, external rotation; elbow extension; forearm neutral.

Working

Arms: Serratus anterior to wrap scapula; anterior deltoid to flex arm; infraspinatus and teres minor to externally rotate at the glenohumeral joint; biceps long head to flex the arm; triceps to extend the elbow; coracobrachialis and pectoralis major to flex and adduct the arm.

Gravity moves the weight of the body deeper into the position, but to do the pose safely, the body is not just passively releasing into gravity. Thus, most of the muscles listed as lengthening are also in some way working at length (eccentrically) to stabilize the pose. In addition, some muscles are working concentrically.

Spine: Concentrically: extensors of the spine. Eccentrically: all the muscles listed as lengthening.

Legs: Front leg: hamstrings, gluteus maximus, gastrocnemius, and soleus, eccentrically; articularis genus, maybe quadriceps, concentrically. Back leg: psoas major, iliacus, rectus femoris, sartorius, and tensor fascia lata, eccentrically.

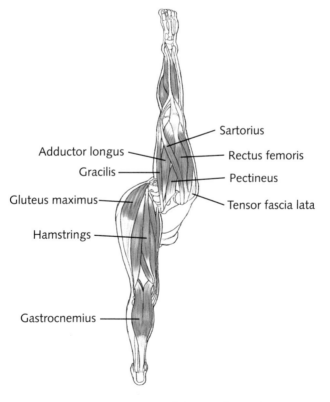

Hanumanasana viewed from underneath.

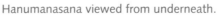

(continued)

Lengthening

Spine: Obliques, psoas minor, rectus abdominis, intercostals in front of the rib cage, anterior longus colli and verticalis, suprahyoid and infrahyoid muscles.

Legs: Front leg: hamstrings, gluteus maximus, piriformis, obturator internus and gemelli, posterior fibers of gluteus medius and minimus, gastrocnemius, and soleus (perhaps other rotators such as quadratus femoris and obturator externus). Back leg: psoas major, iliacus, rectus femoris, sartorius, tensor fascia lata, pectineus, adductor longus and brevis, gracilis (the more internally rotated the back leg, the less vulnerable the adductors are to being strained, as in a "pulled groin muscle").

Obstacles and Notes

In this difficult pose, the forward-bending action in the front leg/pelvic half combines with the backward-bending action in the back leg/pelvic half to create the challenge of keeping the spine balanced between those two contradictory actions.

Because of the opposing action of the legs and pelvic halves, the forward-bending aspect of this pose is more difficult than a forward bend done with both legs, and vice versa. This is due to the opposition action of the other leg, which prevents the spine from doing the flexing or extending. Thus, all the movement in the lower half of the body must come from the sacroiliac joint, hip, and leg.

Because there is generally more hip range of motion in flexion than in extension, the movement of the back leg draws the spine into extension. This is also why more work is often felt in the extensors of the front leg than in the flexors of the back leg.

In a way, this is a bound pose because of the way the action in each leg is limited by the opposite leg. It is therefore possible to overmobilize vulnerable areas (hamstring attachments are especially at risk in this pose). This concern is greatly compounded if the pose is done passively.

If hanumanasana is done more actively, with attention to the eccentric action of the lengthening muscles, the "stretch" of the pose can be distributed over several joints—stabilizing the mobile ones and mobilizing the fixated areas. Neuromuscularly, this eccentric activity also stimulates the muscles' spindle portion of the stretch reflex to release the muscles into greater length. Active use of the antagonistic muscles (for example, contracting the quadriceps) can also activate the "reciprocal innervation" stretch reflex, which stimulates the hamstrings to release further.

In this pose, many people allow the back leg to externally rotate to get it "all the way down." Letting the back leg roll out puts twisting pressure into the lumbar spine and/or the sacroiliac joint of the back leg—not to mention a twisting pressure into the back knee. It also puts more pressure into the adductors of the back leg (longus, brevis, pectineus, and gracilis) without the eccentric support of the iliacus and psoas major or rectus femoris. As a result, the groin gets over-stretched, and the usually overtight rectus femoris doesn't get as much stretch as it could. It's much more rigorous to do this correctly, and much safer for the legs and pelvis.

Breathing

You'll know you're doing this pose effectively when you can breathe freely. Until all the flexion, extension, and rotational forces have been neutralized, and the spine can extend easily, the breathing will tend to be labored and rough. The use of props such as blocks, straps, or blankets is highly recommended so that the work can be done in a gradual way that doesn't excessively disturb the rhythm of the breath.

Kurmasana

Turtle Pose

koor-MAHS-anna

kurma = tortoise, turtle

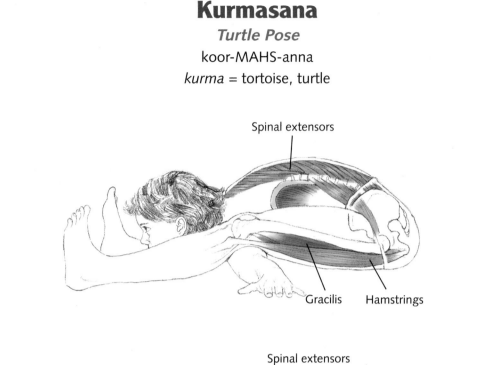

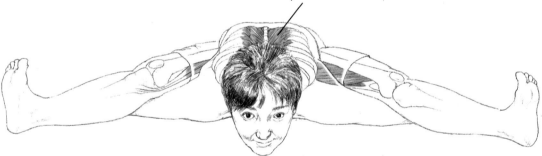

Classification and Level

Advanced seated forward bend

Joint Actions

Cervical extension; thoracic and lumbar flexion, moving toward extension; sacroiliac nutation; hip flexion, abduction, neutral rotation; knee extension; ankle dorsiflexion; scapula elevation, downward rotation, and abduction, moving toward adduction and lateral rotation; glenohumeral joint lateral abduction and internal rotation; elbow extension; forearm pronation.

Working

Gravity pulls the torso toward the floor.

Spinal extensors can act to deepen hip flexion against the resistance of the arms. The extension of the spine presses the arms in this position against the legs, flexing the hips and knees, so the hamstrings activate to extend the hips. The vastii also extend the knees.

The rhomboids and trapezius activate to adduct the scapulae; the posterior deltoids press the arms against the legs; and the biceps resist hyperextension in the elbows.

Lengthening

Legs (similar to upavistha konasana): The piriformis and gluteus maximus are working eccentrically because they are extensors of the hip; the obturator externus and quadratus femoris are working eccentrically because they are also adductors. Of the adductors, the gracilis is especially stretched because of the knee extension; the pectineus is not affected because of the hip flexion. In the hamstrings, the semitendinosus and semimembranosus are particularly lengthened here because of the abduction of the legs.

Spine: Extensors of the spine are lengthening, but active. As the pose deepens, it moves toward more thoracic extension. Spinal extensors lengthen to enter into the pose, then activate. Similarly, the rhomboids lengthen to get into the pose, then contract to reposition the scapulae.

Obstacles and Notes

To prepare for this pose, the spine flexes, the scapulae abduct, and the hips and knees flex. Once the arms are in position under the legs, the actions that deepen the pose are the reversal of the preparatory ones: spinal extension, scapula adduction, and knee extension.

This opposition of actions in the spine and scapulae mean that muscles such as the spinal extensors and rhomboids are asked to contract from a very lengthened position (one of the more challenging positions from which to concentrically contract a muscle).

Because the arms are "bound" under the legs, there is the potential for forcing the action into vulnerable spots: The spine could overflex in the lumbar or thoracic regions, or the hamstrings could overstretch at their attachment on the sitting bones.

Breathing

The diaphragm receives considerable compression when entering into this position, and the gradual movement out of thoracic flexion can be seen as an attempt to reestablish the breathing space in the thoracic cavity.

(continued)

Kurmasana Variation

Supta Kurmasana

Reclining Turtle Pose

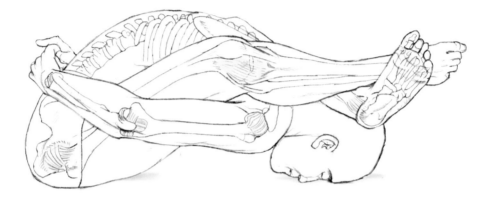

Joint capsules are shaded in blue.

Classification and Level

Advanced seated forward bend

Joint Actions

Full spinal flexion; sacroiliac nutation; hip flexion, external rotation, adduction; knee flexion; ankle dorsiflexion; scapula downward rotation, abduction; glenohumeral internal rotation, extension, adduction; elbow flexion; forearm—left in pronation, right in supination.

Working

Gravity, and the tensegrity of the posture, which is bound.

To enter the pose, spinal flexors (psoas major, rectus abdominis, obliques internal and external) are activated.

Legs: Adductor longus and brevis to externally rotate, flex, and adduct, with help from the obturator externus and quadratus femoris (of the rotators, the ones that do the most adduction).

Arms: Subscapularis, to internally rotate the humerus; pectoralis minor, to downwardly rotate the scapulae; teres major, to internally rotate and extend the arm; posterior deltoid, to extend the arm; triceps long head, to extend the arm.

Lengthening

Hamstrings, gluteus maximus (due to deep hip flexion); gluteus medius and minimus (due to hip adduction); piriformis, obturator internus, gemelli (due to hip flexion and adduction); adductor magnus (due to external hip rotation and flexion).

All spinal extensors are lengthening.

The anterior deltoids, coracobrachialis, and pectoralis major (due to the extension of the arms); trapezius and rhomboids (due to the abduction of the scapulae).

Obstacles and Notes

Using the latissimus dorsi to help internally rotate and extend the arms will interfere with the flexion of the spine, because the latissimus dorsi are also spinal extensors.

This pose has the potential for directing too much force into the spine, sacroiliac joint, and, with the arms bound in this position, the front of the shoulder joint. The subscapularis is working to both internally rotate the humerus and protect the joint from protraction.

The more freedom there is in the scapulae gliding on the rib cage, the less force will be directed into the glenohumeral joint and its capsule.

The bound position of the legs behind the skull and cervical spine creates potential stress in this area, too—either overstretching the back of the neck or overworking the muscles against the push of the legs.

If there isn't enough mobility in the rest of the spine, the cervical spine can be overflexed to get the legs in position. This should be avoided.

Breathing

Good luck. Actually, once locked into this bound pose, the abdominal muscles don't have much to do, so they can be released for good old belly breaths. This is actually advisable, because excessive abdominal action during trunk flexion can stress an already vulnerable neck.

Mahamudra

The Great Seal

ma-ha-MOO-dra

maha = great, mighty, strong

mudra = sealing, shutting, closing

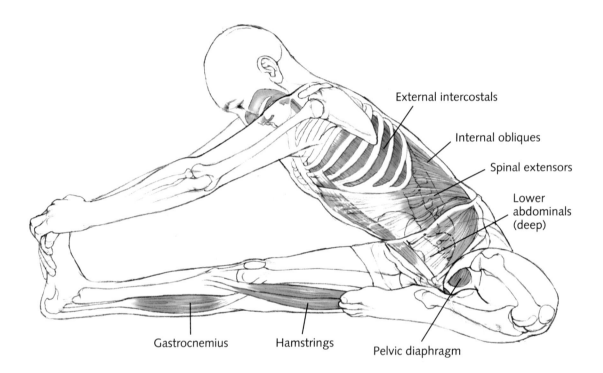

External intercostals

Internal obliques

Spinal extensors

Lower abdominals (deep)

Gastrocnemius　　Hamstrings　　Pelvic diaphragm

Classification and Level

Advanced seated pose for breath practice

Joint Actions

Spine: atlanto-occipital joint flexion; strong axial extension; mild axial rotation in the thoracic spine (necessitated by the turning of the pelvis). Extended leg: hip flexion, adduction, internal rotation; knee extension; ankle is pulled into dorsiflexion. Folded leg: hip flexion, abduction, external rotation; knee flexion; ankle plantarflexion; foot supination. Shoulders and arms: scapula upward rotation, slight abduction, elevation; glenohumeral flexion and adduction; elbow extension; forearm pronation; wrist neutral extension; hand and finger flexion working against the pressure of the foot.

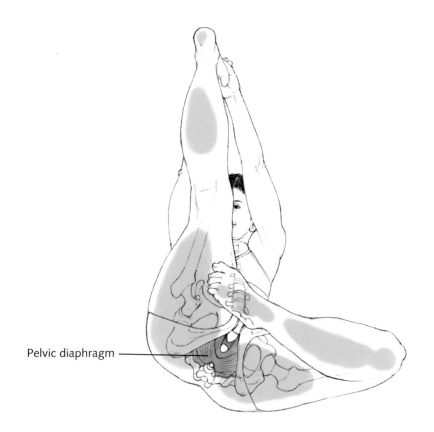

Pelvic diaphragm

Blue areas show the base of support.

Working

Spine: Extensors against the pull of gravity into flexion. Extended-leg-side internal obliques and folded-leg-side external obliques act together to rotate the spine to face the extended leg; the folded-leg-side rotatores and multifidi act to rotate the spine toward the extended leg.

Bandhas: Mula (root lock): deep, lower abdominal muscles (internal obliques, transversus abdominis) and pelvic diaphragm (levator ani, coccygeus). Uddiyana (rib cage lift): external intercostals and costal fibers of the diaphragm (to maintain the circumference at the base of the rib cage) and scalenes for lifting the sternum. Jalandhara (chin lock): sternocleidomastoids bilaterally to flex skull on spine.

Legs: At this angle, gravity acts to flex the hips (as opposed to the vertical of dandasana). The psoas major and iliacus can act to deepen and stabilize the hip flexion.

Extended leg: The adductor magnus and pectineus act to internally rotate and adduct the leg; the vastii work to extend the knee (hopefully without the rectus femoris, whose action would create congestion in the hip in this position).

(continued)

Folded leg: Gravity acts to nutate the sacrum and flex the hip. The obturator externus, quadratus femoris, piriformis, obturator internus, and gemelli externally rotate the hip; the sartorius externally rotates and flexes the hip and knee; the hamstrings act to flex the knee; the tibialis anterior flexes the ankle and supinates the foot.

Arms: The serratus anterior upwardly rotates the scapula; the anterior deltoid and pectoralis major flex and adduct the arms; the triceps extend the elbow; flexor digitorum superficialis, profundus, lumbricals in the hand grasp the toes.

Lengthening

Spine: posterior suboccipitals (eccentrically), sternocleidomastoid.

Extended leg: Hamstrings, gluteus maximus, piriformis, obturator internus, gemelli, some gluteus medius and minimus, gastrocnemius, soleus. Working at length (eccentrically), the popliteus moves the back of the knee toward the floor.

Folded leg: The adductor magnus mainly stretches because it creates internal rotation, extension, and adduction (as in baddha konasana). The adductor longus and brevis also stretch because they flex and externally rotate the leg (abduction lengthens these two). There also might be some lengthening in the tensor fascia lata, because of the external rotation, and in the fibers of the gluteus medius and minimus with increasing hip flexion.

Arms: The rhomboids lengthen, as do the lower trapezius and latissimus dorsi.

Obstacles and Notes

The base of mahamudra is very similar to janu sirsasana, which it resembles. The similarity ends there, however, because the main action of this pose is strong axial spinal extension, which in turn arises from a deep application of the three bandhas (mula bandha, uddiyana bandha, and jalandhara bandha).

A simplified way of thinking about this position is that it combines a forward bend (flexion of the lumbar and cervical spine), a backward bend (extension of the thoracic spine), and a twist (axial rotation of the thoracic spine and the turning of the pelvis toward the extended leg).

A lack of flexibility in any of the structures listed earlier in the "Lengthening" section will lead to excessive action in the "Working" muscles. This will lead to the expenditure of too much energy and the demand for too much oxygen—which will make it impossible to maintain the bandhas.

Breathing

Executing this pose properly while engaging all three bandhas is considered to be the ultimate test of the breath. The reason for this is that mahamudra freezes all the normal respiratory movements out of the body cavities: There is strong stabilizing action in the pelvic floor and abdominal muscles, the rib cage is held in a lifted position, the costovertebral joints are immobilized by thoracic twisting, and the sternum is lifted into the chin by the scalenes. All in all, the body is forced to find another, unusual way to breathe.

When all the usual, visible, external breath movements have been stabilized, something deep in the core of the system must mobilize via a new pathway. That pathway is commonly referred to in yogic literature as susumna—the central channel.

Navasana

Boat Pose

nah-VAHS-anna

nava = boat

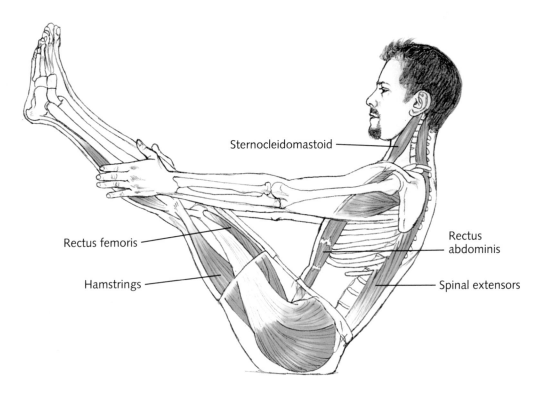

Sternocleidomastoid

Rectus femoris

Hamstrings

Rectus abdominis

Spinal extensors

Classification and Level

Basic seated balance—abdominal strengthener

Joint Actions

Spine neutral extension, resisting flexion; sacroiliac joint neutral, resisting counternutation; hip flexion, adduction, internal rotation; knee extension; ankle neutral extension; scapula neutral (if arms extended to shoulder height); glenohumeral joint flexion, lateral adduction, slight external rotation; forearm neutral rotation.

Working

Spine: The psoas major and spinal extensors work to maintain neutral alignment against the pull of gravity; the abdominal muscles work eccentrically to resist the hyperextension of the lumbar spine. The abdominal muscles also resist the bulging forward of the abdominal organs, which bear the weight of the thorax and arms.

Legs: The psoas major and iliacus flex the hips; the rectus femoris flexes the hips and extends the knees; the vastii extend the knees; the gracilis and pectineus adduct and flex the hip joints; the tensor fascia latae support flexion and internal rotation; the sartorius supports flexion at the hip joints.

Arms: The serratus anterior and rhomboids hold the scapulae on the rib cage; the infraspinatus and teres minor externally rotate the head of the humerus; the coracobrachialis and anterior deltoids flex and laterally adduct at the glenohumeral joints; the triceps and anconeus extend the elbows.

Lengthening

Hamstrings.

Variation with arms extended.

Obstacles and Notes

In this pose the challenge is not the position itself, so much as its relationship to gravity. If it were rotated 45 degrees, it would just be the work of sitting vertically in dandasana (which can certainly present its own challenges).

Ideally, the weight in this pose is distributed between the sitting bones and the tailbone. All the weight should not be borne on the sacrum, because that would create a destabilizing counternutation in the sacroiliac joints.

If dandasana is a challenge because of tight hamstrings, that tightness will make it impossible to support this pose correctly with the legs straight. In this case, bending the knees so the spine can remain neutral is a good option.

It is an interesting challenge to have to work hard to maintain a neutral spine, as opposed to working to get the spine into flexion, extension, or rotation.

This asana is often described as working the abdominal muscles. This is true; however, the abdominal muscles do not hold the weight of the pose. Rather, they are modulators of the action of creating hip flexion, which is mainly performed by the psoas major and iliacus. If the psoas is difficult to access, it is possible to overwork the rectus femoris or tensor fascia latae in this pose.

Just as bending the knees makes this pose easier by shortening the length of the lower lever arm, stretching the arms overhead would make it more difficult by lengthening the upper lever arm.

Breathing

To maintain the stability and balance of this pose, the breath must be very restrained and focused. To illustrate how vital this is, attempt to do navasana while taking deep belly breaths.

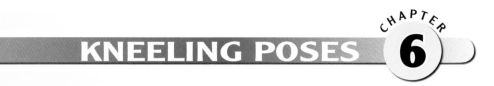
When kneeling, the body's weight is on the knees, shins, and parts of the feet. Kneeling brings the center of gravity closer to the ground and makes certain activities, such as gardening, less stressful for the spine. Without proper care, however, kneeling can be stressful for the knee joints.

This position is also associated with "lowering oneself" in the sense of meekness or worship. This probably evolved from the fact that when kneeling, a person is defenseless and unable to flee. Even the proud, upright stance of kings and pharaohs is tempered by their frequent depiction in this humble position.

In yoga, kneeling poses are often used to help open the hip and knee joints. When the body's weight is taken off the feet and legs, the pelvic muscle attachments can be stretched because they no longer stabilize the body weight high off the ground.

Kneeling also provides a stable base from which the center of gravity can be raised up so the spine can fully extend—most beautifully expressed in poses such as camel (ustrasana) and pigeon (kapotasana).

A position that's frequently used to counterpose strong spinal extensions is child's pose, the kneeling position that produces mild, even spinal flexion and lowers the center of gravity.

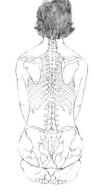

The vajrasana pose.

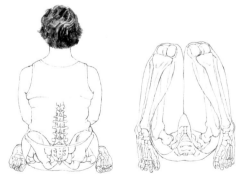

The virasana pose.

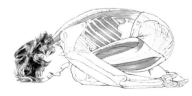

Child's pose.

Supta Virasana

Reclining Hero Pose

soup-tah veer-AHS-anna

supta = reclining, lain down to sleep

vira = a brave or eminent man, hero, chief

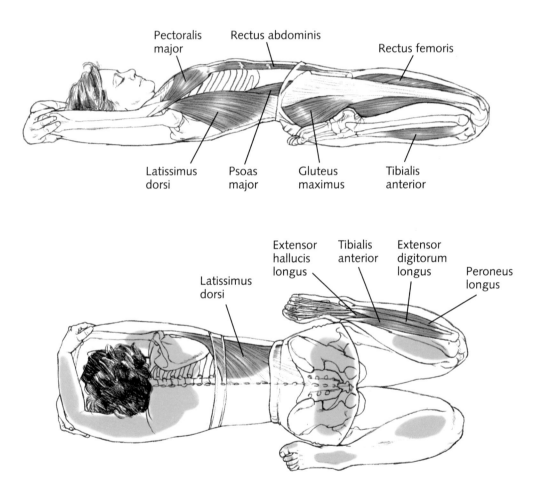

Pectoralis major · Rectus abdominis · Rectus femoris

Latissimus dorsi · Psoas major · Gluteus maximus · Tibialis anterior

Latissimus dorsi · Extensor hallucis longus · Tibialis anterior · Extensor digitorum longus · Peroneus longus

Classification and Level

Intermediate reclining groin stretch

Joint Actions

Spine axial extension (in the full version of the pose); sacroiliac joint counternutation; hip extension, internal rotation, and adduction; knee flexion and tibia medially rotated; ankle plantarflexion; scapula upward rotation, abduction, elevation; glenohumeral joint flexion, external rotation; elbow flexion.

Working

Reclining hero is a released hip opener in which the goal is to relax as much as possible into gravity. The lower abdominal muscles can be activated to prevent hyperextension in the lumbar spine and to lengthen the psoas major.

Lengthening

Rectus abdominis, psoas major (the lower part at first, and the upper part as the pose deepens), iliacus, rectus femoris, sartorius, perhaps the tensor fascia latae, gluteus medius and minimus; vastii, tibialis anterior, extensor digitorum longus, extensor hallucis longus; piriformis, gemelli, and obturator internus (because of internal rotation and adduction); adductor longus and brevis (because of internal rotation and extension); pectineus (because of hip extension).

Obstacles and Notes

There are many variations for the arm position in this pose—at the sides, reaching overhead, and propped up on the elbows (for the less flexible). If the latissimus dorsi are tight, reaching the arms overhead can increase the hyperextension of the spine because of the attachment of the latissimus in the lower back.

Because hip extension in internal rotation is more challenging than in external rotation for most people, supta virasana "forces" the pelvis to be honest about how open the groins truly are. This pose often begins as spinal extension, especially if there is tightness in the hip flexors, because the internal rotation of the legs is bound into place by the weight of the body.

If the hip extensors are tight and the pose is "pushed," the force can be transmitted either into the lower back or into the knees. In either case, the pose should be supported in a way that allows for maximum hip extension; getting down to the floor is less important.

Because the knees are at risk, keeping the feet active and avoiding supination is important for maintaining integrity in the knee joints.

This can be an excellent pose for sciatic and lower-back pain, if done with attention to the internal rotation and extension in the hips. If poorly executed, the pose can exacerbate lower-back pain.

Breathing

The tautness in the psoas and abdominal wall creates both posterior and anterior pressure in the abdominal cavity. This effect is magnified when activating the abdominal muscles to flatten the lumbar curve. The resulting breathing patterns would favor movements above and below the abdominal pressure.

Emphasizing thoracic breath movements at the base of the rib cage helps to mobilize the upper spine and shoulder girdle. Focusing on pelvic floor movements assists in releasing tension in the hips, groin, and gluteal region.

Balasana

Child's Pose, Embryo Pose

BAH-las-anna

bala = young, childish, not fully grown or developed

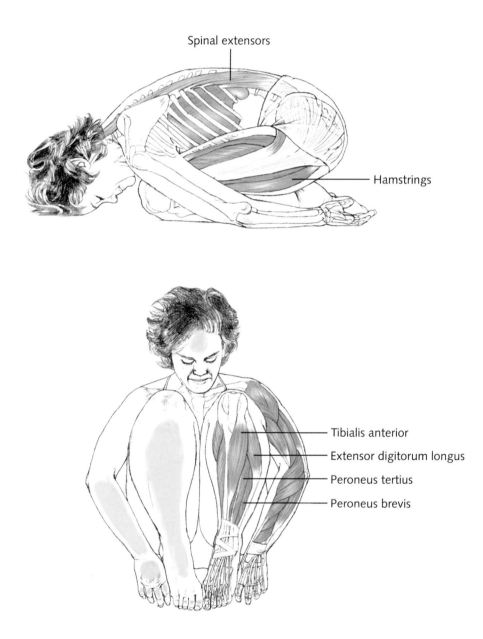

Spinal extensors

Hamstrings

Tibialis anterior

Extensor digitorum longus

Peroneus tertius

Peroneus brevis

Classification and Level

Basic kneeling forward bend

Joint Actions

Full spinal flexion (maybe slight cervical extension, depending on the head position or the length of the neck); hip flexion, neutral rotation, adduction; knee flexion; ankle plantarflexion; scapula abduction and downward rotation; glenohumeral internal rotation; elbow extension; forearm pronation.

Working

Gravity draws the yielding body deeper into this position.

Lengthening

The challenge of this pose is to bring the sitting bones to the heels and the forehead to the floor. To do so, many things have to lengthen: the extensors of the spine, gluteus maximus, piriformis and other rotators, hamstrings, gluteus medius and minimus (because of hip adduction), tibialis anterior, peroneus tertius, extensor digitorum longus and brevis, and extensor hallucis longus and brevis in the feet.

Obstacles and Notes

Variations include widening the knees (hip abduction), which can create more neutral extension in the spine and make room for the belly; extending the arms overhead; clasping the heels with the hands; crossing the arms under the forehead; and turning the head to one side.

Sometimes there is congestion in the front of the hip joints, which can be caused by using the hip flexors to pull the body down toward the thighs, rather than allowing gravity to create that action. The use of props can assist in this release.

Restriction can also be felt in the tops of the feet, if the extensors of the toes are tight or if there is a lack of mobility in the bones of the foot. Additionally, weakness in the intrinsic muscles of the foot will often result in cramping in this, and similar positions (such as virasana and vajrasana).

Breathing

With the hips fully flexed, or adducted, and the front of the torso resting on the anterior surface of the thighs, the movement of the breath in the abdomen and anterior rib cage is greatly restricted. This necessitates more movement in the back of the waist and rib cage. That's why if there is tightness in those places, this pose can feel suffocating.

Ustrasana

Camel Pose

oosh-TRAHS-anna

ustra = camel

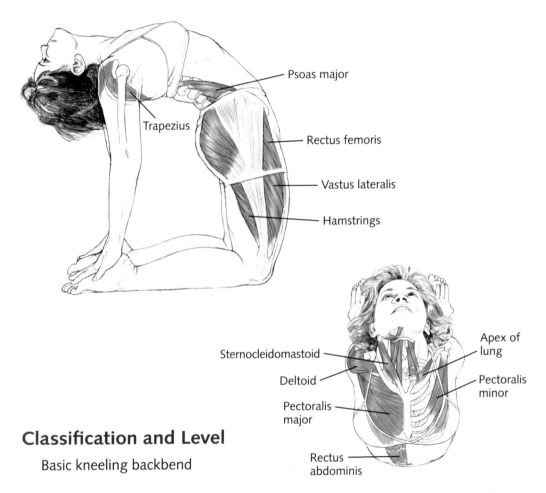

Trapezius

Psoas major

Rectus femoris

Vastus lateralis

Hamstrings

Sternocleidomastoid

Deltoid

Pectoralis major

Apex of lung

Pectoralis minor

Rectus abdominis

Classification and Level

Basic kneeling backbend

Joint Actions

Spinal extension; hip extension and internal rotation; knee extension; scapula downward rotation, adduction, elevation; arm external rotation, extension, adduction; elbow extension.

Working

Gravity is pulling the torso into the backbend, which is checked by the arm action and the eccentric action of the spinal flexors.

Arms: The triceps extend the glenohumeral and elbow joints; the trapezius and rhomboids adduct the scapulae. The posterior deltoids and teres major also extend the glenohumeral joint, while the subscapularis protects it anteriorly.

Spine: In the cervical spine, the anterior neck muscles (longus capitis, longus colli, rectus capitis anterior, suprahyoid, and infrahyoid) work eccentrically to keep the head from collapsing. Also working eccentrically to prevent collapsing into the lumbar spine are the rectus abdominis, obliques (especially external), intercostals, subcostals, iliacus, and psoas major and minor.

Legs: The rectus femoris is working eccentrically against the weight of the pelvis moving backward, and the vastii are working concentrically to press the shins into the floor. The hamstrings and adductor magnus are also working concentrically—mainly to stabilize the knee and hip joints.

Lengthening

Arms: Pectoralis major and minor, coracobrachialis, biceps, and anterior deltoids all stretch.

Spine: In the cervical spine, the anterior neck muscles listed earlier are working at length, but the sternocleidomastoid should be lengthened and relaxed to avoid the base of the skull being pulled into the atlas and axis. The scalenes are also providing support for the anterior spine, as well as the breath (discussed later). In the thoracic region, the internal intercostals are stretched by the opening of the rib cage, as are the scalenes (which are the cranial continuation of the intercostal layers).

Obstacles and Notes

In camel, a mild internal rotation of the legs is recommended to keep the sacroiliac joints stable, which will favor hip and spinal extension over sacroiliac counternutation (which is what happens when this pose is felt "in the small of the back").

It can be very challenging to find a healthy extension of the spine at the base of the neck or the top of the thoracic spine. It helps to focus on releasing the sternocleidomastoid using the eccentric strength of the deeper anterior neck muscles to stabilize the weight of the head. Additionally, in many people, the upper trapezius muscles form a "shelf" in this position that can provide a resting place for some of the weight of the head.

Camel is an intense stretch for the digestive system, especially the esophagus.

Breathing

In ustrasana, the thoracic structures are maintained in an "inhaled" position, and the abdominal wall is stretched. This results in a decreased ability of the body to breathe "normally." The trick is to find support from the deeper musculature so the more superficial efforts can quiet down. Then it's possible to notice an interesting relationship between the deepest layer of superficial neck muscles (scalenes) and the breath movement in the apex of the lungs, which are suspended from the inner scalene muscles.

Eka Pada Rajakapotasana

One-Legged Royal Pigeon Pose

eh-KAH pah-DAH rah-JAH-cop-poh-TAHS-anna

eka = one

pada = foot, leg

raja = king, royal

kapota = dove, pigeon

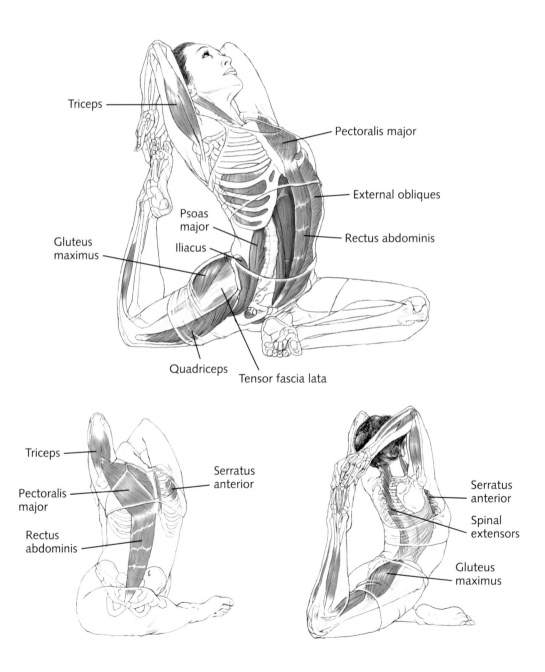

Triceps

Pectoralis major

External obliques

Psoas major

Rectus abdominis

Iliacus

Gluteus maximus

Quadriceps

Tensor fascia lata

Triceps

Serratus anterior

Pectoralis major

Rectus abdominis

Serratus anterior

Spinal extensors

Gluteus maximus

Classification and Level

Advanced kneeling backbend

This pose is categorized with kneeling because that is the starting position, but the base of support is not actually kneeling. This asana has a unique base of support: the back surface of the front leg and the front surface of the back leg. This same base, with the knee joints extended, would be hanumanasana.

Joint Actions

Spinal extension. Front leg: nutation; hip flexion, external rotation, and abduction; knee flexion; ankle and foot supination. Back leg: counternutation; hip extension, internal rotation, and adduction; knee flexion; ankle plantarflexion.

Working

Spine: The spinal extensors work to create the backbend; then the extensors and obliques work to maintain balance and an orientation to the front. The actions in the spine are very similar in this pose to those in natarajasana (see chapter 4), although the action of gravity is slightly different (there is perhaps less anterior tilt to the pelvis, and thus more action in the back hip).

Back leg: Same action as natarajasana; the internal rotation and extension has the joint capsule most taut.

Arms: Same action as natarajasana.

Front leg: Gravity is the main force. The hamstrings, gluteus maximus, and peroneals work eccentrically, pressing into the floor, to keep from collapsing into the pose.

Lengthening

When the front leg is abducted, there is generally less stretch of the rotators, although the obturator externus and quadratus femoris are slightly more lengthened with abduction. More stretch is actually felt in the hamstrings, in spite of the knee flexion.

When the front leg is adducted, the action of flexion and adduction at the hip lengthens the piriformis, obturator internus, and gemelli mainly—and the obturator externus and quadratus femoris slightly less.

When the knee is more extended in the front leg (toward 90 degrees of flexion), the rotation at the hip is greatly intensified. This action may be felt in the gluteus medius and minimus, and/or in the adductor magnus or adductor longus. This action puts more pressure into the knee, especially if there is restriction in the hip joint, and the knee is much more vulnerable to twisting forces when at 90 degrees. The action in the feet and ankles can help to stabilize and protect the knee.

(continued)

Obstacles and Notes

It is important not to collapse into this pose. The pelvic floor, hamstrings, and gluteals should act eccentrically to distribute the weight force of gravity through the whole base of the pose rather than drop right into the hamstring attachment or knee joint.

As with all poses, and more so with complex ones, a wide variety of experiences are available, depending on each person's strength, balance, and range of motion.

Variation

Folded Forward

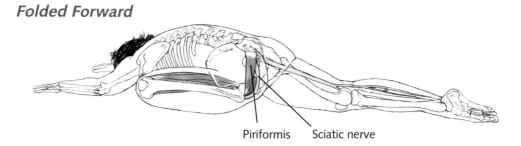

Piriformis   Sciatic nerve

This variation intensifies the action in the hamstrings of the front leg because of deeper hip flexion and more body weight over the front leg. At the same time, it diminishes the action in the back hip and in the spine. By adducting the front leg, the piriformis is brought into the lengthening action.

This is perhaps the most frequently used stretch for the infamous piriformis. Because this muscle crosses over the largest nerve in the body, the sciatic nerve, tightness in this muscle can be a cause of sciatic pain. This variation of pigeon pose helps to release tension in the piriformis in a mostly passive, relaxed position, as opposed to the more active base required of the full pigeon. Being a deep hip stabilizer, the piriformis requires at least a minute of sustained stretching to release its *spindle reflex* and actually begin lengthening. Before the release of the spindles, the main sensation is actually of the muscles *resisting* the stretch to protect themselves from injury. When viewing this pose from underneath, you can see clearly that the sciatic nerve is also stretched in this position.

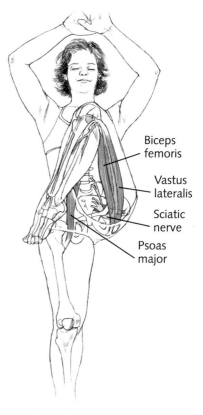

Biceps femoris

Vastus lateralis

Sciatic nerve

Psoas major

Folded forward variation.

The following illustrations show the relationship of the sciatic nerve to the piriformis muscle in the following:

1. Neutral hip position (figure *a*).
2. External rotation and abduction, which actually shortens the piriformis (figure *b*).
3. Hip flexion, which begins the stretch of the piriformis and other external rotators (figure *c*).
4. Hip flexion combined with adduction, which puts the piriformis into maximal stretch, along with the sciatic nerve (figure *d*).

When entering this stretch from the kneeling position, the hip joint is already in flexion. It is then externally rotated as it's brought into maximal flexion, and then moved into adduction before the body's weight is placed on it. As mentioned previously, extending the knee joint to 90 degrees greatly increases the torque on the hip joint, and thus the stretch to the rotators, but poses greater risk to the knee joint.

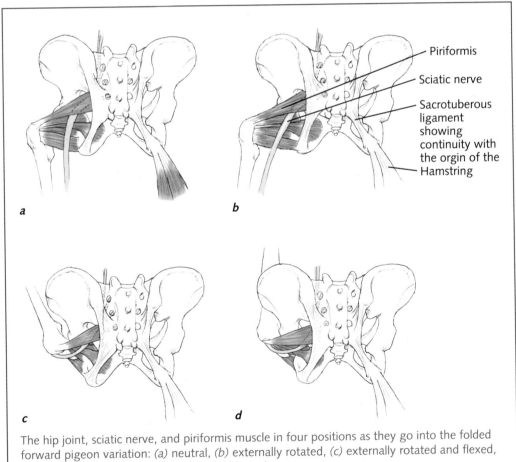

The hip joint, sciatic nerve, and piriformis muscle in four positions as they go into the folded forward pigeon variation: *(a)* neutral, *(b)* externally rotated, *(c)* externally rotated and flexed, and *(d)* externally rotated, flexed, and adducted.

Parighasana

Gate-Latch Pose

par-ee-GOSS-anna

parigha = an iron bar used for locking a gate

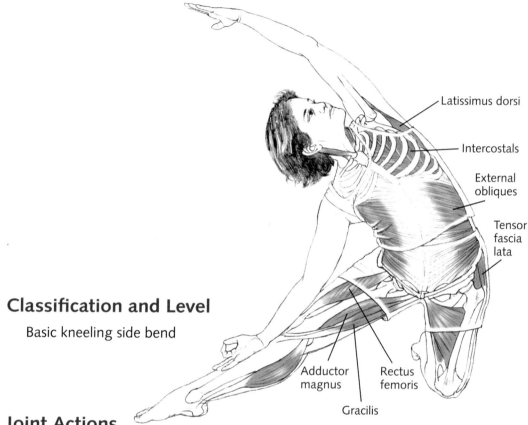

Latissimus dorsi

Intercostals

External obliques

Tensor fascia lata

Rectus femoris

Adductor magnus

Gracilis

Classification and Level

Basic kneeling side bend

Joint Actions

Spine lateral flexion (some rotation to maintain neutral alignment), cervical rotation and extension, sacroiliac neutral. Standing leg: hip neutral extension, adduction, internal rotation; knee flexion; ankle dorsiflexion (to press into the floor for balance). Extended leg: hip flexion, external rotation, abduction; knee extension; ankle plantarflexion. Top arm: scapula upward rotation, elevation; glenohumeral joint external rotation, elevation, flexion; elbow extension; forearm supination. Bottom arm: neutral scapula; glenohumeral external rotation; forearm supination.

Working

Spine: Gravity works on the weight of the torso to pull it toward the floor, so the upper (long side) lengthens eccentrically in the external obliques. Also, to resist the front of the body twisting toward the extended leg, the upper-side internal obliques and lower-side external obliques work concentrically.

Legs: Extended leg: sartorius, piriformis, gemelli, and obturator internus are active to rotate and abduct the leg; the hamstrings and piriformis work to keep from collapsing into the hip joint and/or hyperextending the knee; the soleus and intrinsic muscles of the foot point the toes to the floor. Kneeling leg: gluteus medius and minimus work eccentrically to keep the hip from shifting too laterally; the adductor magnus maintains internal rotation and hip extension, and the quadriceps extend the knee to press the lower leg into the floor for balance, along with the dorsiflexors of the ankle.

Arms: Top arm: serratus anterior to abduct and upwardly rotate the scapula; infraspinatus and teres minor to externally rotate the glenohumeral joint; deltoids to elevate the arm. The lower arm is mostly at rest.

Lengthening

Top side: Rhomboids, latissimus dorsi, long head of triceps, intercostals, quadratus lumborum, external and internal obliques, gluteus medius and minimus, tensor fascia latae, gluteus maximus, rectus femoris, iliacus, and psoas on the standing leg.

Extended leg: Hamstrings, gracilis, adductor magnus.

Obstacles and Notes

Rotation is automatic with side bending in the spine because of both the shape of the articular facets in the vertebrae and the spiral pathways of the muscles. To keep the action "pure" lateral flexion, there needs to be a counterrotation in the rib cage. In this case, the upper ribs rotate posteriorly and the lower ribs rotate anteriorly. To achieve this, the internal obliques on the upper side and the external obliques on the lower side are recruited.

Also, if there is tightness in the outside of the standing leg hip joint (in the tensor fascia lata, gluteus medius, or gluteus minimus), then that hip will try to flex rather than stay purely adducted. The standing leg should maintain hip extension (via the adductor magnus and hamstrings) to prevent this.

When there is tightness in the latissimus dorsi, lifting the arm overhead can push the rib cage forward (compressing the floating ribs and inhibiting breath in general), or pull the scapula downward even as the arm is lifting—potentially creating impingement of the biceps tendon or supraspinatus at the acromion process. Folding the upper arm behind the back eliminates this concern and allows the focus to remain on the torso movement.

Breathing

Which side of the diaphragm moves more in this pose—the upper, stretched side, or the lower, compressed side? Is the answer the same for both sides of your body? Explore.

Simhasana

Lion Pose

sim-HAHS-annah

simha = lion

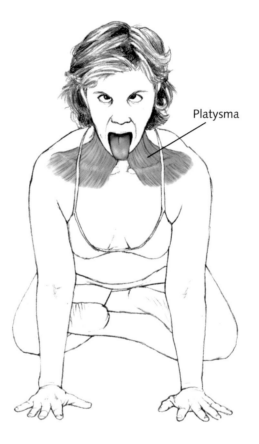

Platysma

Classification and Level

Basic kneeling jaw stretch

Joint Actions

Atlanto-occipital joint flexion; spine neutral extension; adduction and elevation of the eyeballs.

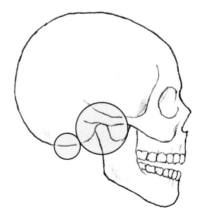

The temporomandibular joint represents the center of gravity of the skull, while the atlanto-occipital joint is its base of support.

Working

The lengthening activation of the tongue lifts the hyoid bone; activates the digestive system; and activates the hyoid muscles, sternum, rectus abdominis, pubic bone, and pelvic floor.

A strong exhalation (lion's roar) activates the three diaphragms: thoracic, pelvic, and vocal. The platysma muscle can also be contracted in simhasana. The superior and medial rectus muscles of the eye both contract to direct the gaze inward and upward.

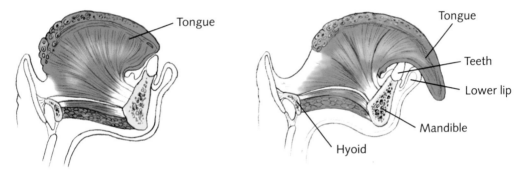

Tongue extension.

Stretching

Jaw muscles: temporalis, masseter, lateral and medial pterygoids, tongue.

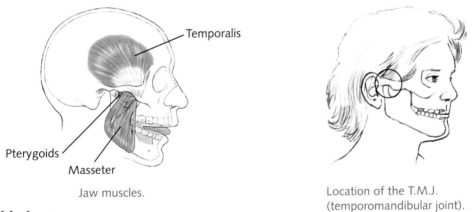

Jaw muscles.

Location of the T.M.J. (temporomandibular joint).

Notes

Simhasana stimulates and releases a host of oft-overlooked muscles. The tongue and jaw can be thought of as the front of the neck, and cervical tension can frequently be related to tightness in these structures. Additionally, the platysma (the flat, thin, rectangular muscle that covers the front of the throat) can be tonified during simhasana. Aside from the cosmetic advantages (a weak platysma is associated with wrinkly throat skin), consciously contracting this muscle increases the ability to relax it during inspiratory efforts.

As a variation, this pose can also be done from kneeling.

SUPINE POSES

Supine means lying in a faceup position. It is the opposite of prone, which is lying facedown. Similarly, *supination* means to turn a hand, foot, or limb upward, whereas *pronation* refers to turning them downward.

Both words originate in Latin: *Supinus* means "leaning backward," and *pronus* means "leaning forward." Interestingly, this is the reverse of what's possible from each position. From a supine position, only forward movement (spinal flexion) is possible; from a prone position, only backward movement (spinal extension) is possible.

Just as tadasana and samasthiti are the quintessential standing positions, savasana is the prototypical supine position. In the corpse pose, the back surface of the body becomes the base of support, and all the postural muscles can relax from their constant dance with gravity.

Savasana has the lowest center of gravity and is the starting point of all the supine poses. It is also the position in which those asanas usually end. Because no effort is required to stabilize the body while it is supine, poses that evolve from here are—by definition—mostly langhana (see page 16) and become more brahmana as the center of gravity is raised higher.

Moving into postures from a supine position engages the anterior musculature of the body, which is why many abdominal strengthening exercises start in this position.

Savasana

Corpse Pose

shah-VAHS-anna

sava = corpse

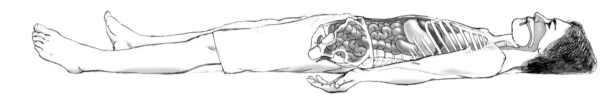

Occasionally, this pose is referred to as the death pose, or mrtasana (mrit-TAHS-anna). *Mrta* means death.

Classification and Level

Depending on the perspective, either very easy or very advanced

Working

Gravity and mental focus.

The corpse pose is said to be the easiest asana to perform, but the hardest to master. Whatever gymnastics demands the other asanas may make to your balance, strength, or flexibility, the challenge of completely releasing the tension from every part of the body and mind is perhaps the greatest test of the yogi.

Anatomy

Primary and Secondary Curves

In savasana, the structures that are in full, weight-bearing contact with the floor exhibit the primary curves of the body (see chapter 2). These include the posterior surfaces of the calcaneus, gastocnemius, hamstrings, gluteus maximus, sacrum, thoracic spine, scapulae, and occiput.

The structures that are off the floor mirror the secondary curves of the body—specifically, the posterior surfaces of the Achilles tendons, knee joints, lumbar region, and cervical spine.

The point of contact of the arms varies widely from person to person, depending on the unique shape and relationships of the upper-body structures—particularly the elbow joint.

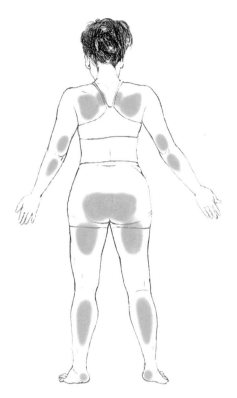

Blue areas show the weight-bearing structures, including the primary curves.

Symmetry

Many people never fully relax in savasana because of an obsession with arranging the body in a perfectly symmetrical shape, which they verify visually, but which conflicts with the body's kinesthetic (proprioceptive) feedback. In other words, what *looks* symmetrical is not what *feels* symmetrical.

Because all human bodies are inherently asymmetrical, a certain amount of surrender to this fact is necessary to achieve a deep state of emotional, as well as physical, relaxation. If you want to fully relax, you need to accept your body as it is, not as you would wish it to be.

Breathing

A deep state of conscious relaxation is quite different from sleep, which is a common experience in this pose. In savasana, the body is completely at rest and its metabolism is freed of the demands of contending with gravity, making it possible to practice the most difficult breathing exercise of all: the act of being fully aware of—but not controlling—the breath's movements.

Normally, when you are aware of your breathing, in some way you alter its natural rhythm. When you are not aware of the breath, it is driven by a combination of autonomic impulses and unconscious habit. The juxtaposition of active awareness and surrender to the breath's natural movements makes possible the powerful realization that true surrender is an act of will.

Dwi Pada Pitham

Two-Legged Table

dvee PA-da PEET-ham

dwi = two

pada = feet

pitham = stool, seat, chair, bench

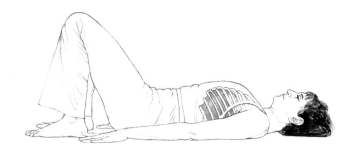

Exhale.

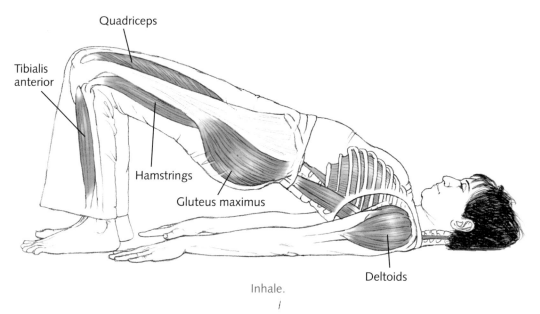

Quadriceps

Tibialis anterior

Hamstrings

Gluteus maximus

Deltoids

Inhale.

Classification and Level

Basic supine vinyasa

Except for the arm position, the muscular, spinal, and joint actions of this pose are virtually identical to those of setu bandhasana (which is described later in this chapter).

The main difference between setu bandhasana and dwi pada pitham is that dwi pada pitham is a *vinyasa*, a dynamic movement that is coordinated with the inhalation and exhalation.

This simple, yet versatile practice can be used in a variety of ways to release tension from the spine and breathing structures, as well as to help balance the leg and hip actions that support similar poses, such as setu bandhasana and upward bow, or wheel (see chapter 9).

Breathing

The lifting movement is typically done on the inhalation and the lowering on the exhalation, but this pattern can be changed to produce various effects. For example, the three bandhas can be very easily activated simply by doing the lowering movement on an external retention (bhaya kumbaka). Lowering the spine on a retention after an exhalation creates a natural lifting of the pelvic floor and abdominal contents toward the zone of lowered pressure in the thoracic cavity. The subsequent inhalation can create a dramatic downward release of the pelvic floor and a noticeable sense of relaxation in this often tense region.

Apanasana

Apana Pose

ap-AN-ahs-anna

apana = the "vital air" that eliminates waste from the system

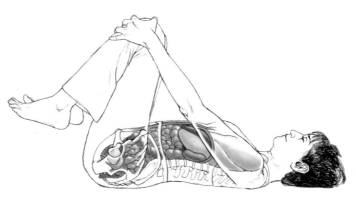

Inhale.

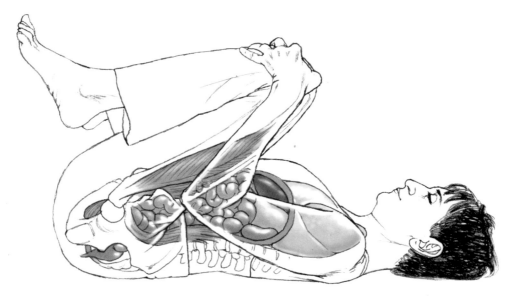

Exhale.

Another simple, yet useful practice that directly links breath and body movement, apanasana is one of the key tools of therapeutic yoga. It stimulates the upward release of the diaphragm on the exhalation, as the knees are drawn into the body. Traditionally this is done by actively using the abdominal and hip flexor muscles without the assistance of the arms, which are just "along for the ride." An interesting difference can be felt if the hip flexors and abdominal muscles are relaxed and the arms are used actively to "pump" the thighs against the abdomen, deepening the exhalation.

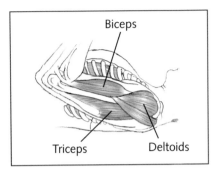

Because so much lower-back tension is the result of a tense diaphragm, apanasana is one of the simplest and most effective ways of helping the lower spine, by creating more diaphragmatic "space" for the abdominal muscles to create postural support.

Taken together, dwi pada pitham and apanasana constitute a powerful pair of counterposing movements that can dramatically reverse some of the most common health complaints.

Viparita Karani

Inverted Pose

vip-par-ee-tah car-AHN-ee

viparita = turned around, reversed, inverted

karani = doing, making, action

Classification and Level

Basic supine inversion

Joint Actions

Spine cervical and upper thoracic flexion; lower thoracic and lumbar extension; hip flexion, adduction, internal rotation; knee extension; ankle neutral extension; scapula adduction, downward rotation, elevation; glenohumeral joint external rotation, extension, adduction; elbow flexion; forearm supination; wrist extension (dorsiflexion).

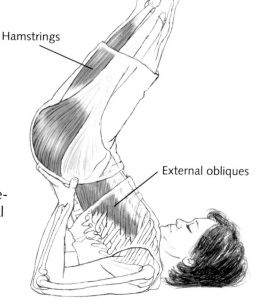

Hamstrings

External obliques

Working

Spine: Psoas minor, obliques, rectus abdominis, and transversus, eccentrically, to resist gravity; the muscles of the anterior rib cage, to resist the weight of the lower body.

Legs: Pectineus, to adduct, flex, and internally rotate the legs; adductor magnus, to adduct and internally rotate; tensor fascia latae may help with internal rotation and flexion; vastii, to extend knees.

Shoulders: Rhomboids, to adduct scapulae; levator scapulae, to elevate scapulae (in this case, press scapulae into the floor) and medially rotate the bottom tips of the scapulae (which tips the glenoid fossa downward); trapezius, to adduct, elevate, and medially rotate the bottom tips of the scapulae. Pectoralis minor is also active to downwardly rotate the scapulae (the more adduction of the scapulae, the less the pectoralis minor can work).

Arms: Infraspinatus and teres minor, to externally rotate the head of the humerus; subscapularis and coracobrachialis, eccentrically, to protect the front of the joint from protraction; long head of triceps and teres major, to extend the shoulder and adduct the arm; posterior deltoid, to extend and externally rotate the arm; biceps brachii and brachialis, to flex the elbow and supinate the forearm; flexor carpi radialis, ulnaris, and flexor digitorum superficialis and profundus, eccentrically, to support the weight of the hips.

Lengthening

Abdominal muscles are lengthening as they are working, eccentrically, the muscles of the anterior rib cage.

Legs: Hamstrings, gastrocnemius, and soleus might feel mild lengthening.

Shoulders: Serratus anterior, coracobrachialis, pectoralis major, possibly pectoralis minor (depending on the angle of the upper rib cage to the scapulae).

Arms: Flexors of the forearm and hand are working eccentrically, lengthening while holding the weight of the pelvis and legs.

Obstacles and Notes

In a shoulder stand, the erector muscles of the spine are more active than in viparita karani. In the "lifted" version of viparita karani, the abdominal muscles play a greater role than the spinal muscles to keep the pelvis from collapsing onto the hands.

In viparita karani the abdominal muscles are strongly active in eccentric contraction. If they do not have the ability to modulate their lengthening, the weight of the pelvis will collapse onto the hands or wrists. Practicing the ability to enter and leave this pose will help with other actions that require abdominal eccentric control—for example, dropping the legs over into the wheel from a headstand or handstand, controlling vrksasana, dropping back into the wheel from tadasana, and so forth.

Body proportions and individual differences in weight distribution between the upper and lower body will greatly affect the experience of this pose. A prime example is how challenging (strengthwise) it can be for women because of the greater proportion of weight in their lower bodies and the greater flexibility of their spines, compared with men (which makes their abdominal muscles work extra hard to stabilize).

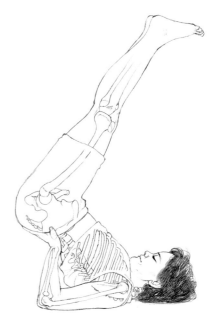

Dropped version of viparita karani.

Breathing

This position offers the opportunity to experience all three bandhas: the lower abdominal action of mula bandha, the opening at the base of the rib cage (supported by the hand position) of uddiyana bandha, and the chin lock associated with cervical flexion known as jalandhara bandha.

The inverted nature of viparita karani produces the cleansing, eliminative effects associated with the upward movement of apana. The supported versions of this pose are a valuable staple of restorative yoga practice.

Salamba Sarvangasana

Supported Shoulder Stand

sah-LOM-bah sar-van-GAHS-anna

salamba = with support (*sa* = with, *alamba* = support)

sarva = all

anga = limb

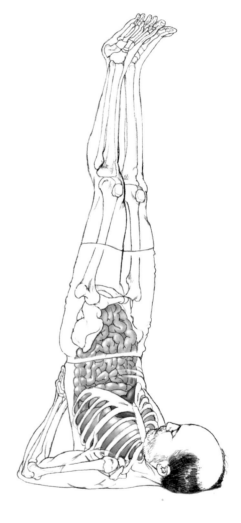

The term *salamba* distinguishes this variation of the shoulder stand from the unsupported (*niralamba*) version.

Classification and Level

Basic supine inversion

Joint Actions

Spine cervical flexion; thoracic flexion; lumbar flexion moving toward neutral extension; sacroiliac joint nutation; hip neutral extension, adduction, neutral rotation; knee extension; ankle neutral extension; scapula adduction, downward rotation, elevation; glenohumeral joint external rotation, extension, adduction; elbow flexion; forearm supination; wrist extension (moving toward flexion as the hands press into the back).

Working

Spine: The intrinsic muscles of the spine (intertransversarii, interspinalis, rotatores, multifidi, spinalis, semispinalis, splenius capitis and cervicis, longissimus, and iliocostalis) are all active in the shoulder stand to keep the legs from falling toward the face. The psoas minor, obliques, rectus abdominis, and transversus are very active in the pose to keep from falling backward.

Working eccentrically in the neck: rectus capitis posterior major and minor, obliquus capitis superior and inferior.

Legs: To maintain a neutral alignment of the legs against the pull of gravity, the adductor magnus and hamstrings hold the legs together and extend the hips. The vastii extend the knees. The medial fibers of the gluteus maximus act to extend the hips (without external rotation).

Shoulders: The rhomboids work to adduct the scapulae; levator scapulae elevate the scapulae (in this case, to press their upper edges into the floor), and also medially rotate the bottom tips of the scapulae (which angles the glenoid fossa downward toward the hips). The trapezius acts to adduct, elevate, and medially rotate the bottom tips of the scapulae. The pectoralis minor is also active to downwardly rotate the scapulae. (Again, the more adduction of the scapulae, the less the pectoralis minor is active.)

Arms: The infraspinatus and teres minor externally rotate the head of the humerus; the subscapularis and coracobrachialis work eccentrically to pro-tect the front of the joint from protraction; the long head of triceps and teres major act to extend the shoulder and adduct the arm; the posterior deltoid works to extend and externally rotate the arm; the biceps bra-chii and brachialis act to flex the elbow and supinate the forearm; the flexor carpi radia-lis, ulnaris, and flexor digitorum superficialis and profundus work to press the hands into the back.

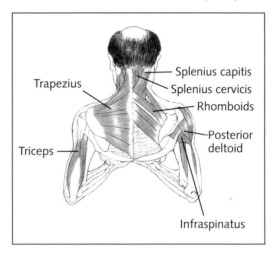

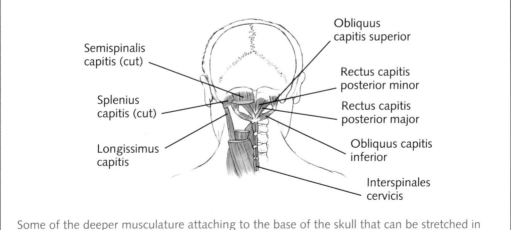

Some of the deeper musculature attaching to the base of the skull that can be stretched in shoulder stand, plow pose, and variations.

(continued)

Salamba Sarvangasana *(continued)*

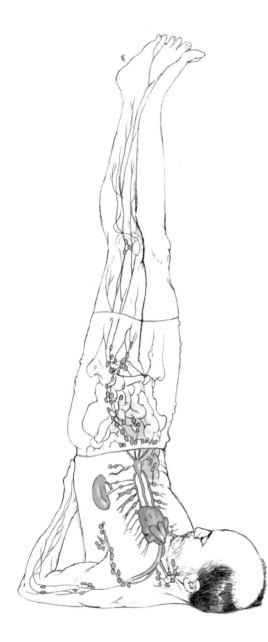

Lymph drainage in shoulder stand.

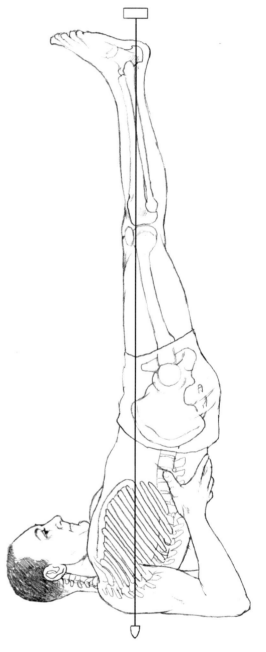

Center line of gravity passing through the base of support.

Lengthening

Muscles of thoracic spine are lengthened at the same time they are taking the weight of the lower thorax and legs.

In the shoulders, the serratus anterior, coracobrachialis, and pectoralis major all lengthen.

Obstacles and Notes

Entering the pose from the plow (halasana) is more demanding on the extensors of the spine, especially the thoracic spine, because they are in an elongated position before contracting. Entering from the bridge pose (setu bandhasana) is more demanding on the extensors of the shoulder joints and the flexors of the spine (the psoas and abdominal muscles).

From the perspective of the muscles of the spine and abdomen, being in this pose is less challenging than getting into it. However, remaining in the pose is more challenging for the muscles of the scapulae, because they are all bearing the static load of the body while either contracting or lengthening.

To truly be a shoulder stand, the muscles that adduct, downwardly rotate, and elevate the scapulae must be strong enough to take the weight of the entire body. If they are not, and the shoulders spread apart, the weight falls too much on the upper thoracic and cervical spine.

Breathing

The more mobility there is in the scapulae (or the less resistance from other muscles of the thorax), the less compromised the breath will be in this position. This pose takes a tremendous amount of both flexibility and strength in the entire shoulder girdle. Without the integrity of the shoulder girdle, the weight collapses down into the thorax, and the diaphragm becomes obstructed.

Keeping the base of the rib cage open allows the diaphragm and abdominal viscera to shift effectively toward the head so the full benefits of inversion can occur.

Niralamba Sarvangasana

Unsupported (No-Arm) Shoulder Stand

neera-LOM-bah sar-van-GAHS-anna

Classification and Level

Intermediate supine inversion

Joint Actions

Spine: Same as described in salamba sarvangasana.

Legs: Same as salamba sarvangasana.

Arms: Scapula adduction and upward rotation, elevation; glenohumeral joint external rotation, neutral flexion, adduction; elbow extension; forearm pronation to neutral; wrist and finger extension to neutral.

Working

Spine: Same as salamba sarvangasana, plus the spinal flexors. The upper fibers of the psoas major and abdominal muscles engage strongly to maintain the position without the support of the arms; eccentrically in the neck—rectus capitis posterior major and minor, and obliquus capitis superior and inferior. Also deep anterior neck muscles—longus colli, longus capitis, and verticalis, to maintain flexion in the cervical and upper thoracic spine.

Legs: Same as salamba sarvangasana.

Shoulders: Rhomboids, to adduct the scapulae; serratus anterior, to upwardly rotate the scapulae (modulated by rhomboids to maintain the adduction of the scapulae); levator scapulae, to elevate the scapulae (in this case, press the scapulae into the floor); trapezius, to adduct and elevate the scapulae.

Quadriceps

Hamstrings

Gluteus maximus

Gluteus medius

Latissimus dorsi

Arms: Infraspinatus and teres minor, to externally rotate the head of the humerus; biceps brachii and anterior deltoids, to flex the arms (the arm position is neutral, but the action is that of flexion against the weight of gravity); triceps, to extend the elbows.

Obstacles and Notes

In this pose, the scapulae are adducted *and* slightly upwardly rotated; without the levering action of the arms, this calls on the muscles that move the scapulae on the rib cage to work strongly, in what can be thought of as a contradictory action. If the scapulae are not maintained in adduction, the weight of the body falls into the spine; if the scapulae do not upwardly rotate, the arms are challenged in reaching to the knees. The scapulae are positioned in neutral rotation as they extend to the knees, but the action that gets them there is upward rotation, as they come from the downward rotation of sarvangasana.

The upper fibers of the psoas major and abdominal muscles are very strongly engaged here to maintain the spinal flexion in the thoracic spine. In addition, more lumbar flexion occurs to bring the legs farther overhead and counterbalance the pull of gravity. Reducing this tendency toward lumbar flexion makes the spinal flexors work much harder eccentrically—against the body weight's tendency to roll down to the floor.

In this balancing act between spinal flexors and extensors, imbalances that are usually imperceptible show up, because the arms aren't available to leverage symmetry. When these torques appear, they make this pose that much more challenging to balance.

Breathing

In niralamba sarvangasana, the intense action in the full-body's flexor and extensor groups creates quite a challenge to the shape change of breathing. Because this is a challenging balance pose that requires a lot of stabilizing action in the abdominal and thoracic musculature, any attempt at deep breathing will destabilize the pose even as the full-body activation of these major muscle groups creates a demand for significant oxygenation.

Efficiency—finding the minimum amount of effort necessary to maintain the position—allows the limited breath movements to supply just enough energy to sustain the pose.

Setu Bandhasana

Bridge Pose

SET-too BAHN-dahs-anna

setu = dam, dike, or bridge

bandha = lock

setubandha = the forming of a causeway or bridge, a dam, or bridge

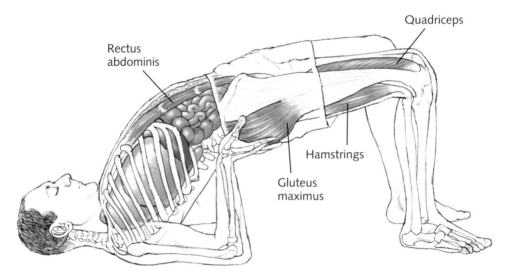

Classification and Level

Basic supine inversion

Joint Actions

Spine cervical and upper thoracic flexion; lower thoracic and lumbar extension; sacrum counternutation; hip extension, adduction, and internal rotation; knee flexion; ankle dorsiflexion; scapula adduction, downward rotation, elevation; glenohumeral joint external rotation, extension, adduction; elbow flexion; forearm supination; wrist extension (dorsiflexion).

Working

Spine: Spinal extensors, especially in the mid- and lower thoracic; psoas minor and abdominal muscles, eccentrically, to prevent overextension in the lumbar spine.

Legs: Hamstrings, to extend the hips and flex the knees, especially the medial hamstrings to adduct and extend the hips; adductor magnus, to extend, internally rotate, and adduct the hips; medial fibers of gluteus maximus, to help extend the hip; tibialis anterior, to dorsiflex the ankle and pull the knees forward; vastii, to extend the knees.

Shoulders: Rhomboids, to adduct the scapulae; levator scapulae, to elevate the scapulae (in this case, press the scapulae into the floor) and medially rotate the bottom tips of the scapulae (which tips the glenoid fossa downward); trapezius, to adduct, elevate, and medially rotate the bottom tips of the scapulae. The pectoralis minor is also active to downwardly rotate the scapulae (the more adduction of the scapulae, the less the pectoralis minor can work).

Arms: Infraspinatus and teres minor, to externally rotate the head of the humerus; subscapularis and coracobrachialis, eccentrically, to protect the front of the joint from protraction; long head of triceps and teres major, to extend the shoulder and adduct the arm; posterior deltoid, to extend and externally rotate the arm; biceps brachii and brachialis, to flex the elbow and supinate the forearm; flexor carpi radialis, ulnaris, and flexor digitorum superficialis and profundus, eccentrically, to support the weight of the hips.

Lengthening

Spine: Psoas minor, rectus abdominis, obliques, anterior rib cage muscles.

Legs: Rectus femoris, psoas major, and iliacus.

Shoulders: Serratus anterior, coracobrachialis, pectoralis major, pectoralis minor.

Arms: Flexors of the forearm and hand are working eccentrically, lengthening while holding the weight of the pelvis and legs.

Obstacles and Notes

It can be a challenge to get full hip extension in this pose. If the hamstrings and adductor magnus are not strong enough, the gluteus maximus may do too much and pull the legs into external rotation; or the other adductors will activate to bring the knees together but also flex the hips; or the rectus femoris will work to extend the knees, but won't fully extend the hips.

Spinal extensors, especially lumbar, may try to help, but too much lumbar extension is not helpful, because it will limit hip extension by putting tension on the psoas complex.

The action in the arms is the same as for the shoulder stand and viparita karani; the action in the hips and legs is the same as for lifting into urdhva dhanurasana.

All in all, considering the many muscle actions that must be balanced for this pose to work, sustaining this basic posture actually requires a high degree of coordination.

Breathing

The three bandhas can be active here, as in viparita karani. The main difference is that in bridge pose, mula bandha must be applied much more actively and against the lengthened resistance of the abdominal wall.

Halasana

Plow Pose

hah-LAHS-anna

hala = plow

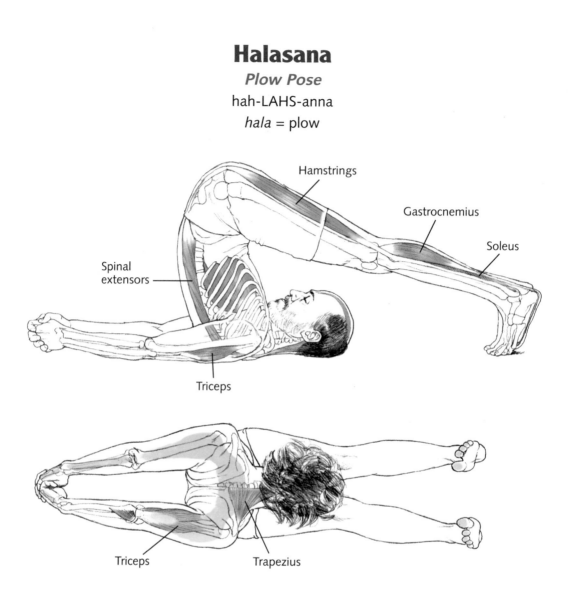

Classification and Level

Basic inverted supine forward bend

Joint Actions

Spine cervical flexion; thoracic flexion; lumbar flexion; sacroiliac joint nutation; hip flexion, adduction, internal rotation; knee extension; ankle dorsiflexion; toe extension; scapula adduction, downward rotation, elevation; glenohumeral joint external rotation, extension, adduction; elbow extension; forearm pronation; wrist extension; finger and hand flexion to clasp hands.

Working

Spine: Similar to sarvangasana, but more active in the intrinsic spinal muscles to keep the spine lengthened.

Working eccentrically in the neck: rectus capitis posterior major and minor, obliquus capitis superior and inferior.

Legs: Gravity, to flex hips; adductor magnus, gracilis, and pectineus, to maintain internal rotation and adduction against the pull of the gluteal muscles; vastii, to extend the knees; tibialis anterior, extensor digitorum, and extensor hallucis, to extend the toes.

Shoulders: Similar to sarvangasana, but working more strongly against the weight of the legs in hip flexion.

Arms: Infraspinatus and teres minor to externally rotate the head of the humerus; subscapularis and coracobrachialis, eccentrically, to protect the front of the shoulder joint from protraction; long head of triceps and teres major to extend the shoulder and adduct the arm; posterior deltoid, to extend and externally rotate the arm; triceps, to extend the elbow; pronators in forearm; flexor carpi radialis, ulnaris, and flexor digitorum superficialis and profundus, to clasp hands.

Lengthening

Spine: Spinal extensors through whole spine.

Legs: Gluteus maximus, hamstrings, gastrocnemius, and soleus.

Shoulders: Serratus anterior, coracobrachialis, pectoralis major, pectoralis minor.

Obstacles and Notes

There are many variations of this pose, some of which have a reputation for being more risky than others. For example, consider the variation of extending the arms overhead and clasping the toes. As in karnapidasana and nirlamba sarvangasana, this upwardly rotates the scapulae and makes the adduction of the scapulae difficult to maintain—the rhomboids and trapezius then lengthen, and weight falls into the upper spine. This variation can overstretch the thoracic and cervical spine, as there is potentially damaging pressure from the pushing action of the feet and, if the hamstrings and gluteals are tight, from the limited hip flexion forcing greater spinal flexion.

Because this pose can produce very intense flexion for the spine, especially the cervical region, it's more important to maintain the integrity of the scapulae and cervical and thoracic spine than to get the legs to the floor—support the legs, if necessary, to protect the neck.

Breathing

As in the shoulder stand, keeping the base of the rib cage open allows the diaphragm and abdominal viscera to shift effectively toward the head, so the full benefits of inversion can occur. This can be much more of a challenge in this pose, because the hip flexion tends to create more intra-abdominal pressure.

Halasana is a very good gauge of how freely you can breathe. It's one thing to have the muscular flexibility to get into the pose, but quite another to have the diaphragm and organs be free enough to remain there and breathe comfortably.

Karnapidasana

Ear-to-Knee Pose

karna-peed-AHS-anna

karna = ear

pidana = squeeze, pressure

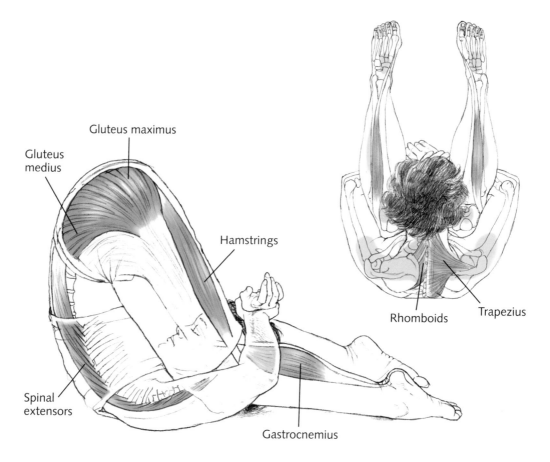

Gluteus maximus

Gluteus medius

Hamstrings

Spinal extensors

Gastrocnemius

Rhomboids

Trapezius

Classification and Level

Intermediate inverted forward bend

Joint Actions

Spinal flexion, hip and knee flexion, scapula abduction and upward rotation, arm flexion, elbow flexion.

Working

Gravity. Slight abdominal and hip flexor action for balance (to keep from rolling backward).

Lengthening

Spine: Extensors of the spine should all lengthen evenly, ensuring that the opening is distributed along the whole spine. Otherwise, the weight of the legs and pelvis can put too much pressure and forced lengthening into the vulnerable muscles of the neck and upper back.

Arms: The rhomboids and trapezius are lengthened here by the abduction of the scapulae and the pressure of the lower body into the upper back.

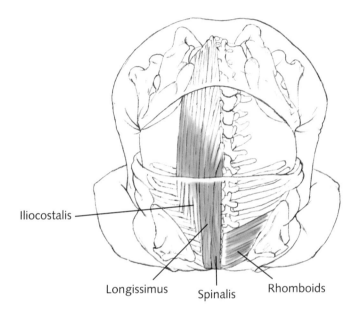

Iliocostalis

Longissimus   Spinalis   Rhomboids

Obstacles and Notes

This counterposes the shoulder action of sarvangasana because the spinal extension and scapular adduction of shoulder stand is reversed, so the muscles that were active are now lengthening. If the release is too passive, however, the muscles can be overstretched.

The support shifts in this pose to the spinous processes of the thoracic spine from the scapulae and trapezius.

Breathing

In ear-to-knee pose, the weight of the lower body is bearing down into the torso, which is in maximal flexion—this is basically, an inverted, weight-bearing exhalation.

The restriction that this position imposes on the breath shouldn't be a problem as long as the body is flexible enough to be in repose. If the muscles are tense, the limited capacity to breathe will soon result in the muscles' inability to fuel their activity; at this point, the asana should be exited.

Jathara Parivrtti

Belly Twist

JAT-hara pari-VRIT-ti

jathara = stomach, belly, abdomen, bowels, or the interior of anything

parivrtti = turning, rolling

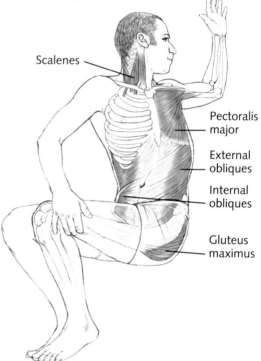

Scalenes

Pectoralis major

External obliques

Internal obliques

Gluteus maximus

Classification and Level

Basic supine twist

Joint Actions

Axial rotation of the spine, hip flexion, knee flexion, scapula resting on rib cage, external rotation in far arm, internal rotation in near arm.

Working

Mostly gravity. The spinal extensors are working somewhat to resist flexion in the lumbar spine.

Lengthening

Top leg: External obliques; intercostals; transversospinalis; gluteus medius, minimus, and maximus; piriformis; gemelli; and obturator internus.

Bottom leg: Internal obliques, intercostals, oblique muscles of erector spinae.

Side of neck the head is turned toward: Sternocleidomastoid.

Side of neck the head is turned away from: Capitis posterior, obliquus capitis inferior, splenius capitis, rectus capitis anterior, scalenes.

Arm the head is turned toward: Pectoralis major and minor, coracobrachialis, latissimus dorsi, brachial plexus nerve bundle.

Notes

As this asana's name would indicate, the belly region of the body is the focus of this twist; therefore, many people assume that this twist arises from the lumbar spine. This is incorrect, however, because the lumbar spine is extremely limited in axial rotation (5 degrees total). The first joint above the sacrum that is capable of significant twisting is T11-T12, and that is where the opposition of the rib cage to the pelvis begins.

To ensure that this twist is evenly distributed throughout the spine, it is important to maintain a neutral spine. This is a challenge with both knees bent, because it's much easier to move into lumbar flexion to deepen the rotation. However, this puts pressure into the lumbar vertebrae and discs, as well as loading the T11-T12 disc. Another challenge to the neutral spine is that tightness in the lateral line will pull the spine into extension, lifting the far shoulder off the floor and compressing the brachial plexus. This often results in sensations of numbness or tingling in the arm.

Breathing

Because the body is supported by the floor, and the main action is provided by gravity, the breathing and postural muscles are free to release in jathara parivrtti. The breath can thus be directed in various ways to achieve specific effects. Bringing the breath movements to the abdomen, for example, will release the tone in the abdominal wall and pelvic floor and assist in reducing extraneous muscle tension in the lumbar region. The opposite pattern of restraining the abdominal wall during the inhalation (mula bandha) will direct the action of the diaphragm into the thoracic structures, mobilizing the costovertebral joints. A similar effect can be achieved in the seated twists (see the discussion of ardha matsyendrasana in chapter 5).

Variation

Belly Twist With Legs Extended

Top leg hamstrings are lengthening. Tightness there can contribute to spinal flexion. The bottom leg's hamstrings are active and help counter spinal flexion with extensor action.

With the bottom leg extended, there is more adduction of the top leg and possibly more internal rotation, which leads to increased length in the iliotibial band; gluteus minimus, medius, and maximus; piriformis; gemelli; and obturator internus.

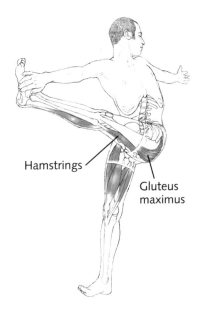

Hamstrings

Gluteus maximus

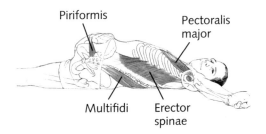

Piriformis

Pectoralis major

Multifidi

Erector spinae

Matsyasana

Fish Pose

mots-YAHS-anna

matsya = fish

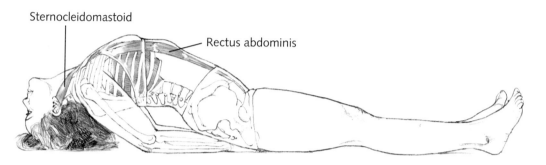

Sternocleidomastoid

Rectus abdominis

Classification and Level

Basic supine backbend

Joint Actions

Spine extension; mild hip flexion, adduction, internal rotation; knee extension; scapula downward rotation, adduction; glenohumeral joint extension, adduction, internal rotation; elbow flexion; forearm pronation.

Working

Spine: Spinal extensors, psoas major (especially lower fibers).

Legs: Psoas major, iliacus, pectineus, tensor fascia latae; hamstrings, to ground legs; quadriceps, for hip flexion and knee extension.

Arms: Shoulder joint: subscapularis, to internally rotate; teres major, to internally rotate; latissimus dorsi, to internally rotate and extend; triceps long head, to extend the shoulder. Trapezius and rhomboids adduct the scapulae; pronators in the forearm turn the hands toward the floor.

Lengthening

Anterior neck muscles; anterior rib cage expands (internal intercostals); the abdominal muscles lengthen, but work eccentrically to resist the anterior displacement of the organs caused by the psoas pushing them forward; in the arms, coracobrachialis and pectorals lengthen, along with the long head of the biceps, serratus anterior, and anterior deltoids.

Obstacles and Notes

This pose can be done while focusing on using spinal extensors (which include the psoas major on the front of the spine) or supported on the elbows. If the support of the elbows is used, there is less work in the muscles of the torso and perhaps more ease in breathing and more expansion.

If the pose is done while focusing on the muscles that extend the spine, the neck will be better protected when lifting the arms off the floor. Variations can also be done with blocks under the spine, and with the feet in baddha konasana (see chapter 5) or padmasana.

This pose is a great demonstration of the role of the psoas major in both hip flexion and spinal extension.

Fish pose is frequently used as an immediate counterpose to the shoulder stand because it reverses the position of the cervical spine from extreme flexion to extreme extension. However, going from one static extreme to the other may not be the most beneficial way to compensate for the stresses of the shoulder stand. A more therapeutic approach would be to gradually reverse the movement of the neck with simple vinyasas leading up to cobra pose (bhujangasana; see chapter 8).

Breathing

In fish pose, the chest is expanded, but not as maximally as in the more difficult arm-supported urdhva dhanurasana. As a result, there is still room for the inhaling action to further expand the rib cage, using the arms as leverage.

Variation

Fish Pose With Arms and Legs Lifted

Joint Actions

Spinal extension; hip flexion, adduction, internal rotation; knee extension; scapula upward rotation, abduction; glenohumeral joint flexion, adduction, external rotation; and elbow extension.

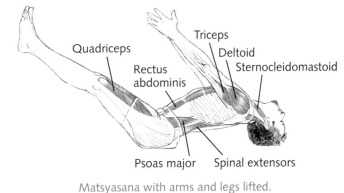

Matsyasana with arms and legs lifted.

Working

Legs: Greatly increased action in the legs when lifted off the floor—especially the psoas major, iliacus, and rectus femoris.

Arms: With the change in arm position, the coracobrachialis, no longer lengthening, is now working to flex and adduct the arm; as are the pectorals and anterior deltoids. The serratus anterior is recruited to abduct the scapulae, and the triceps are extending the elbow.

For a more calming effect—particularly if using the matsyasana as a counterpose—a focus on gentle abdominal breathing can be quite useful.

Anantasana

Reclining Vishnu Couch Pose

anan-TAHS-anna

ananta = endless, eternal (*anta* = end, *an* = without)

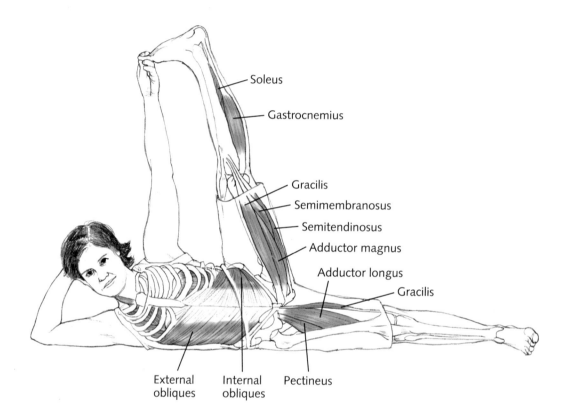

- Soleus
- Gastrocnemius
- Gracilis
- Semimembranosus
- Semitendinosus
- Adductor magnus
- Adductor longus
- Gracilis
- External obliques
- Internal obliques
- Pectineus

Ananta is also the name given to the mythical serpent that the god Vishnu reclines on like a couch.

Classification and Level

Easy side-lying pose

Joint Actions

Spine neutral curves, lateral flexion. Lifted leg: sacrum nutation; hip flexion, external rotation, and abduction; knee extension; ankle dorsiflexion. Bottom leg: hip neutral extension, internal rotation, adduction; knee extension; ankle dorsiflexion; and foot eversion for balance.

Working

Spine: If the left leg is lifted, the left internal and right external obliques are active to resist twisting.

Top leg: Piriformis, obturator internus, and gemelli, to externally rotate and abduct; gluteus medius and minimus posterior fibers, to abduct the leg; quadriceps, to extend the knee; iliacus, to flex the hip.

Bottom leg: Hamstrings active to resist hip flexion (translated from the top leg); the gluteus medius and minimus work to stabilize the leg on the pelvis and the leg to the floor; the adductor magnus acts to counter the gluteus medius and minimus, to keep the pelvis as level as possible.

Lengthening

Top leg: Hamstrings, adductor magnus, gracilis, pectineus (of the adductor group, these are the most lengthened).

Bottom leg: Adductor longus and brevis, gracilis.

Obstacles and Notes

Generally, when the leg is lifted, the pelvis and lower body twist backward. The challenge is to find the counteraction deep in the pelvis rather than through rotating the spine. The gluteus maximus and rotators can be used in the bottom leg to stabilize the pelvic half only if that bottom leg is well grounded.

Breathing

Anantasana is one of the few true side-lying poses. In side lying, the dome of the diaphragm closest to the floor moves cranially (toward the head), while the other dome moves caudally (toward the tail). This is due mainly to the effect of gravity on the abdominal organs, which are pulled toward the floor, taking the diaphragm with them. In addition, the lung closest to the floor (the dependent lung) becomes more supported, and its tissue becomes more compliant, meaning that it's under less mechanical tension and responds more easily to the action of the diaphragm.

Consciously creating this asymmetry in the respiratory mechanism can be useful in breaking up deeply ingrained breathing habits. For example, this pose can be beneficial to people trying to change the habit of sleeping on only one side of the body.

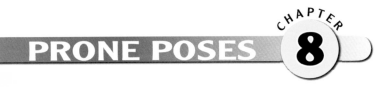
Prone means lying in a facedown position. Moving into postures from a prone position engages the posterior musculature of the body, which is why many back-strengthening exercises start in this position.

Because of the pressure that the prone position puts on the spinal curves, particularly the cervical region, it is not comfortable to remain prone for extended periods of time, and it is not a recommended sleeping position for this reason.

There are only a few backward-bending poses that begin in the prone position, and they are usually counterposed by entering into the kneeling pose of the child.

Socially, this position has even more of a connotation of surrender than kneeling. In many religious traditions, placing the entire front surface of the body on the floor is known as a full prostration.

Bhujangasana

Cobra Pose

boo-jang-GAHS-anna

bhujanga = serpent

(*bhuja* = arm or shoulder + *anga* = limb)

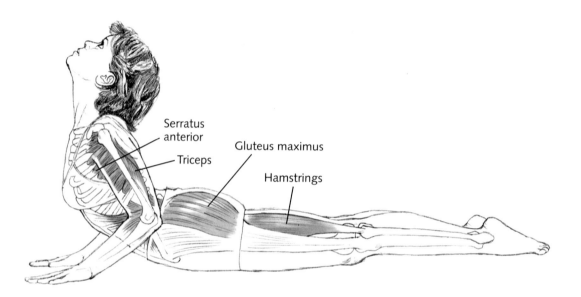

Serratus anterior

Triceps

Gluteus maximus

Hamstrings

Classification and Level

Basic prone backbending pose

Joint Actions

Spine extension; sacrum counternutation; hip extension, internal rotation, adduction; knee extension; ankle plantarflexion; scapula neutral (possibly upward rotation); glenohumeral joint external rotation; elbow extension; forearm pronation.

Working

Spine: The entire spinal extensor group—intertransversarii, interspinalis, rotatores, multifidi, spinalis, semispinalis, splenius capitis and cervicis, longissimus, iliocostalis—work concentrically to create extension. In addition, there is strong action in the serratus posterior superior, which assists chest expansion and synergizes the action of the erectors, which it overlays. The rectus abdominis and obliques work eccentrically to prevent overmobilization of the lumbar spine.

Arms: Infraspinatus, teres minor, serratus anterior, posterior deltoids, triceps, pronator teres, pronator quadratus.

Legs: Many people assume the legs should be passive in cobra, but numerous actions in the legs are required to keep the joints in alignment. The hamstrings, especially semitendinosus and semimembranosus, extend the hips and maintain adduction and internal rotation. The extensor portion of the adductor magnus, along with the deep and medial fibers of the gluteus maximus, also extend the hips without externally rotating the legs. The vastus lateralis, medialis, and intermedius work to extend the knees. Weakness in the medial hamstrings can cause the gluteus maximus to do more than its share of hip extension, in which case the legs will externally rotate, abduct, or both.

Lengthening

Spine: Rectus abdominis, obliques, external intercostals, longus colli and capitis, suprahyoid, infrahyoid, scalenes, anterior longitudinal ligament.

Arms: Latissimus dorsi, teres major, pectoralis major and minor, biceps, and supinators.

Legs: Rectus femoris, lower fibers of psoas and iliacus, and tensor fascia latae.

Obstacles and Notes

It is important to find the deeper intrinsic back muscles to do the action of spinal extension in this pose. Using the latissimus dorsi and other more superficial muscles will affect the scapulae and rib cage and interfere with breathing by inhibiting the movement of the ribs.

In cobra, the serratus anterior is active to maintain a neutral position of the scapulae against the push of the arms. When the arms push, the shoulders don't elevate, but the spine is lifted.

The latissimus dorsi are not helpful as extensors of the spine, because they create flexion of the upper back and internal rotation in the arms.

Weakness in the pronators of the forearm, or tightness in the supinators (or interosseus membrane), will make the elbows flare out to the side and will affect both the elbow and shoulder joints. The forearms should stay parallel to each other for the best alignment of action through the arms into the spine.

(continued)

Breathing

Although the standard instruction is to inhale while entering into a backbend, it can be very helpful to enter into this basic backbend on an exhalation. For many people who are locked into a "belly breathing" pattern, their inhalation will actually restrict thoracic extension and rib cage expansion (this is because a belly breath is accomplished by restricting rib movement while the diaphragm contracts).

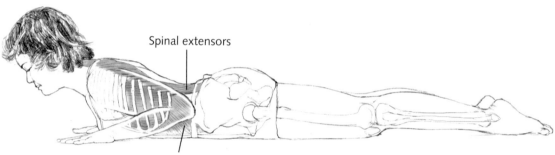

Spinal extensors

External obliques

Variation

Cobra With Knees Flexed

In this position, the hamstrings are used for both actions: hip extension and knee flexion. This position of the leg puts the hamstrings at a very short working length, which greatly increases the chances of cramping in the muscles.

This position also makes it more likely that the outer fibers of the gluteus maximus will fire to help with the hip extension, which will also externally rotate and abduct the legs. Often, a student who can keep the legs adducted and parallel when the knees are extended will find it much more challenging when the knees are flexed. In this position, all of the quadriceps are lengthened, and the stretch in the rectus femoris can restrict the range of motion in knee flexion, too.

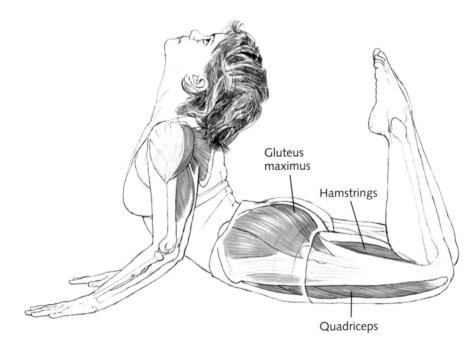

Gluteus maximus

Hamstrings

Quadriceps

Cobra variation with knees flexed.

Dhanurasana

Bow Pose

don-your-AHS-anna

dhanu = bow

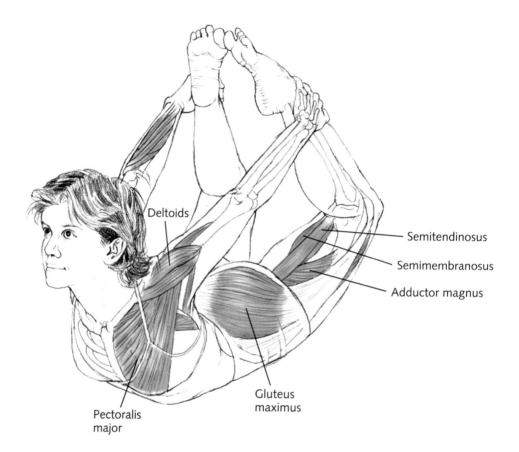

Deltoids

Semitendinosus

Semimembranosus

Adductor magnus

Gluteus maximus

Pectoralis major

Classification and Level

Basic or intermediate prone backbend

Joint Actions

Spine extension; sacrum counternutation; hip extension, medial rotation, adduction; knee flexion; ankle plantarflexion; scapula adduction, elevation; glenohumeral joint medial rotation, extension, adduction; elbow extension; forearm pronation; finger and hand flexion.

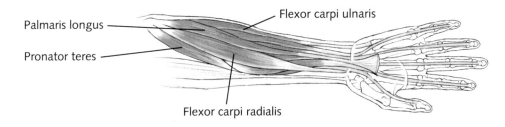

Palmaris longus

Pronator teres

Flexor carpi ulnaris

Flexor carpi radialis

Working

Arms: Working to stabilize arm and scapula position are the subscapularis, teres major, posterior deltoids, rhomboids, levator scapulae, and triceps. Eccentrically working in the opposite direction as they lengthen are the pectoralis major and minor, coracobrachialis, anterior deltoids, and serratus anterior.

Legs: Working to extend the hip joints are the hamstrings, especially semitendinosus and semimembranosus, the extensor portion of adductor magnus, and the deep and medial fibers of gluteus maximus. The vastus lateralis, medialis, and intermedius, and the lower part of the rectus femoris are working to extend the knees.

Lengthening

Legs: Because of hip extension, the rectus femoris, the lower fibers of the psoas, the iliacus, and possibly the pectineus and tensor fascia latae.

Notes

The front of the shoulder joint is structurally vulnerable in this position. If the scapulae are not mobilized in the direction of the stretch (adduction, elevation), too much pressure could be put into the anterior glenohumeral joint, resulting in an overstretch of the subscapularis or damage to the joint capsule. Because this is a bound pose, the pressure into these vulnerable joints is greater.

This pose can be "worked" in a variety of ways by emphasizing different actions: by deepening the action in the spine, by increasing hip extension, or by using knee extension to deepen spine and hip extension. The balance of actions in the hip and knee will be affected depending on whether the hamstrings or the quadriceps are more activated. Because this is a bound pose, with the hands grasping the ankles, it is possible to put too much pressure into the knees. Thus, the alignment of the leg at the hip and the activation of the feet are important to maintain the integrity of the knee.

Breathing

It is a common practice to rock back and forth in this pose by pushing the belly into the floor with each inhalation. It is less common (but much more intense) to practice *not* rocking by directing the inhalation into the already expanded chest region.

Salabhasana

Locust Pose

sha-la-BAHS-anna

salabha = grasshopper, locust

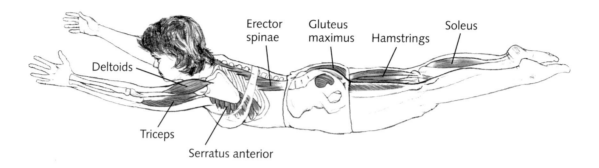

Classification and Level

Basic symmetrical backward bend (although there are asymmetric variations)

Joint Actions

Spine extension; sacrum counternutation; hip extension, medial rotation,
adduction; knee extension; ankle plantarflexion; scapula upward rotation,
elevation, abduction; glenohumeral joint external rotation, flexion; elbow
extension; forearm neutral; wrist neutral.

Working

Arms: Working to lift the arms are the supraspinatus, long head of the biceps
brachii, triceps, anterior and medial deltoids, serratus anterior, and the
trapezius.

Spine: Working to extend the spine are the spinal extensor group: intertransversarii, interspinalis, rotatores, multifidi, spinalis, semispinalis, splenius
capitis and cervicis, longissimus, iliocostalis.

Legs: Working to extend the hips are the hamstrings (semimembranosus,
semitendinosus, and biceps femoris) and the deep, medial fibers of gluteus
maximus. The adductor magnus are active to keep the knees together, and
keeping the knees extended are the vastus lateralis, medialis, and intermedius. The soleus is active to point the foot.

Lengthening

Latissimus dorsi, pectoralis minor, rhomboids, long head of triceps, rectus abdominis; because of hip extension: rectus femoris, iliacus, and lower psoas.

Obstacles and Notes

It can be a challenge to lift the arms in this relationship to gravity, with the spine in extension. If the latissimus dorsi are used to extend the spine (rather than the deeper, intrinsic spinal muscles), they will inhibit the movement in the arms.

This position of the legs uses a complex interaction among adductors, medial rotators, and hip extensors. This is because many of the muscle actions that lift and support the body in this position create other actions that must be neutralized by opposing or synergistic muscles. For example, because the gluteus maximus, a powerful hip extensor, also externally rotates the legs, it's preferable to use the hamstrings for hip extension. Additionally, the gluteus medius and minimus, which help with internal rotation, also happen to abduct the leg, so the adductors will kick in to keep the legs together. Therefore, there are always lots of synergistic actions going on. People will have different priorities, or challenges, depending on where they start and their preexisting patterns of strength/weakness and flexibility/tightness.

Breathing

To rock, or not to rock? All the weight of the body is brought to bear on the abdomen in this variation of locust. While holding the pose for several breaths, the body will rock back and forth with the action of the diaphragm if the primary breathing pattern is "belly breath." An interesting challenge is to keep from rocking, which necessitates a release in the thoracic structures and diaphragm, allowing the floor to push into the abdomen, rather than the abdomen pushing into the floor.

Viparita Salabhasana

Full Locust Pose

vip-par-ee-tah sha-la-BAHS-anna

viparita = reversed, inverted

salabha = grasshopper, locust

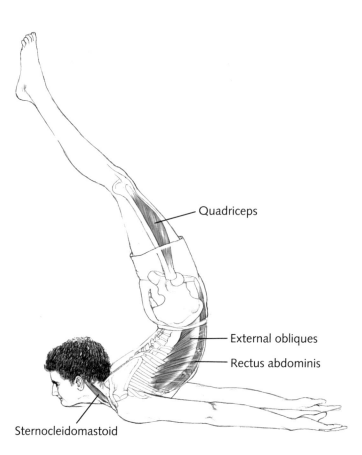

Quadriceps

External obliques

Rectus abdominis

Sternocleidomastoid

Classification and Level

Advanced symmetrical backward bend

Joint Actions

Spine extension, sacrum counternutation; hip extension, medial rotation, adduction; knee extension; ankle plantarflexion; scapula downward rotation, elevation, abduction; glenohumeral joint external rotation, flexion, adduction; elbow extension; forearm neutral; wrist neutral.

Entering Pose:

Working

Concentrically: hamstrings, gluteus maximus, spinal extensors, flexors of glenohumeral joint (pectoralis major, anterior deltoid, biceps, coracobrachialis, serratus anterior). Eccentrically: subscapularis, to protect the glenohumeral joint.

Remaining in Pose:

Working and Lengthening

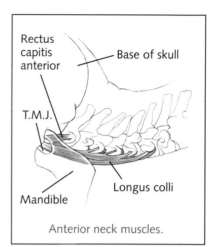

Anterior neck muscles.

Eccentrically: vastii, obliques, rectus abdominis, and anterior neck muscles (longus colli, longus capitis, rectus capitis anterior, suprahyoid, infrahyoid, scalenes, sternocleidomastoid), thoracic diaphragm.

Notes

From the previous analysis of muscular actions, it's clear that what it takes to get into this pose is almost completely the opposite of what it takes to remain in it. Lifting the weight of the body into spinal extension requires a strong, integrated action of the arms and spinal extensors. Once past vertical, gravity will pull the weight of the body into extension, so the trunk flexors must kick in to prevent hyperextension. Therefore, based on their balance of strength and flexibility in the extensor and flexor muscle groups, some people may have the ability to get into full locust, but not to sustain it; whereas others can't get there themselves, but can stay there if assisted into the pose.

Breathing

The standard instruction to inhale while entering into a backbend can be counterproductive here. This is because a strong contraction of the diaphragm will draw the base of the rib cage and lumbar spine (the diaphragm's origin) toward the central tendon (its insertion). This can create considerable resistance to the lengthening in the deep front line of the body. Exhaling while lifting the body into the pose works better for many people.

Remaining in the pose requires the abdominal wall to remain tautly active, which can limit abdominal breath movement, while the actions that synergize the push of the arms into the floor tend to limit thoracic excursion. In addition, having the neck in weight-bearing extension can add resistance to the airway, not to mention that all of this is happening in an inverted position. All in all, this is a very challenging position to breathe in. Efficiency of effort is the key.

ARM SUPPORT POSES

In spite of their obvious similarities, the upper and lower extremities of the human body have evolved to perform specific functions. The structure of the foot, knee, hip, and pelvis points to their function of support and locomotion.

The highly mobile structures of the hand, elbow, and shoulder girdle are clearly ill-suited to weight bearing. In fact, if you compare the proportional structure of the hand and foot, you will see a completely inverse relationship between the weight-bearing and articular structures within them.

In the foot, the heavy, dense tarsal bones comprise half the length of its structure. Adding to this the weight-bearing function of the metatarsals, it can be said that four fifths of the foot's structure is dedicated to weight bearing. The foot's phalangeal structures contribute only one fifth of its total length.

These proportions are completely reversed in the hand, where half the length of the structure is composed of the highly mobile phalangeal bones. The hand's metacarpals are also very mobile (compared to the metatarsals), whereas the relatively immobile carpals (wrist bones) comprise only one fifth of the total length of the hand. This means that, even if you effectively recruit the metacarpals in arm support, you still have only half the length of the hand available for weight bearing.

The bottom line is that when you use the hand in weight-bearing poses, you have to respect the fact that it is at a structural disadvantage. You must therefore compensate for this fact when you prepare for and execute such poses.

In modern Western culture, many people overuse and misuse their arms and hands while working at computers. This is why all the arm supports in this book are categorized as intermediate or advanced; beginning students don't put weight on their hands until they've fully experienced standing on their feet.

Adho Mukha Svanasana

Downward-Facing Dog Pose

AH-doh MOO-kah shvah-NAHS-anna

adho mukha = having the face downward

shvana = dog

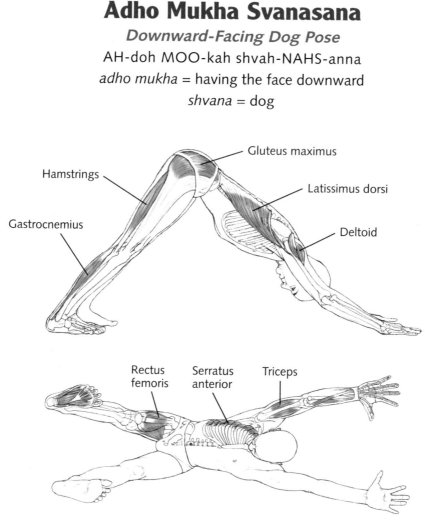

Classification and Level

Intermediate inverted arm support

Joint Actions

There are many approaches to working with this pose. Fundamentally, it is a great opportunity to observe the effects of the arms and legs on the spine.

Assuming the spine is in neutral, or axial extension, then you move toward flexion in both the glenohumeral (shoulder) joint and the hip joint and toward extension in the elbow and knee.

Spine neutral or axial extension; scapula upward rotation and elevation, initially abducted, but advanced students move toward adduction; glenohumeral joint flexion and external rotation; elbow extension; forearm pronation and wrist extension; sacrum nutation; hip flexion (with perhaps some internal rotation); knee extension; ankle dorsiflexion.

Working

Spine: Psoas minor, obliques; deep extensors work very precisely to maintain neutral spinal alignment (axial extension).

Legs: Working against gravity. If the hamstrings are tight, the hip flexors (iliacus, rectus femoris, pectineus) may activate to assist with hip flexion, but this is not actually desirable. The adductor magnus internally rotates and moves the femur back. To extend the knee, the vastii and articularis genus activate. To deepen the dorsiflexion in the ankle, the intrinsic foot muscles need to maintain the integrity of the arches of the foot, so the extrinsic muscles can release in the ankle.

Arms: Also working against gravity. The serratus anterior upwardly rotates and abducts the scapulae, while the infraspinatus, teres minor, and posterior deltoids work to externally rotate the glenohumeral joints. Because the flexion of the glenohumeral joints is created by gravity, the anterior deltoids can relax.

To extend the elbow and resist collapse in the shoulder, the triceps are active. The latissimus dorsi often try to help this action, but they depress and internally rotate the shoulder, which creates impingement at the acromion process.

The pronators are active in the forearm, but if there is lack of rotation between the radius and ulna, this can translate into overarticulation in the elbow or wrist, or internal rotation of the arm at the shoulder joint—all common sites of injury for practitioners of vinyasa styles of yoga that employ repetitive downward-facing dogs in sun salutations.

As in the foot and leg, the intrinsic action in the hand is essential for the integration of the whole arm. Essentially, the hand must act as much as a foot as possible by maintaining its arch. The flexor carpi radialis and ulnaris should activate to resist the collapse of the hand.

Lengthening

Spine: Diaphragm, intercostals.

Legs: Hamstrings, gastrocnemius, soleus, gluteus maximus. Release is needed in the psoas major, iliacus, rectus femoris, tibialis anterior, tensor fascia latae, and pectineus.

Arms: Latissimus dorsi and teres major are lengthening. The long head of the triceps is working eccentrically (at length).

Breathing

From the perspective of the breath, downward-facing dog is an inversion with the spine in axial extension. Because inversions naturally move the diaphragm cranially, the exhaling action of the abdominal muscles can be quite deep. If the lower abdominal action is maintained when initiating the inhalation (mula bandha), the thoracic structures will be encouraged to mobilize, which can be quite challenging in an arm support pose.

Urdhva Mukha Svanasana

Upward-Facing Dog Pose

OORD-vah MOO-kah shvon-AHS-anna

urdhva = rising or tending upward, raised, elevated

mukha = face

shvana = dog

Classification and Level

Intermediate backbending arm support

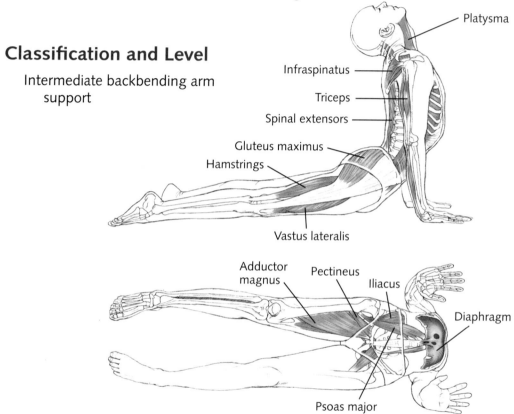

Platysma

Infraspinatus

Triceps

Spinal extensors

Gluteus maximus

Hamstrings

Vastus lateralis

Adductor magnus

Pectineus

Iliacus

Diaphragm

Psoas major

Joint Actions

Full spinal extension; sacroiliac counternutation; hip extension, internal rotation, and adduction; knee extension; ankle plantarflexion; toe extension; scapula adduction, upward rotation; glenohumeral joint extension, neutral rotation (to maintain neutral shoulder alignment, some people need to internally rotate and some people need to externally rotate the humerus); elbow extension; forearm pronation; wrist extension; finger extension.

Working

Spine: Throughout the spine, the extensors are active, though mostly in the thoracic spine. Gravity creates much of the extension in the lumbar spine, so the psoas minor is active eccentrically to resist too much lumbar lordosis, and the obliques do the same. In the cervical spine, gravity, acting on the weight of the head, creates extension, so the anterior neck muscles work eccentrically to keep the action balanced. In the thoracic spine, the semispinalis thoracis, the spinalis thoracis, the thoracic part of the interspinalis, and the rotatores are most active in deepening the thoracic extension.

Legs: To extend the hips, the hamstrings work along with the extensor portion of the gluteus maximus. The adductor magnus internally rotates, extends, and adducts the hip joints, and the gracilis helps with adduction. The vastii and articularis genus work to extend the knees.

Arms: The serratus anterior upwardly rotates the scapulae in synergy with the rhomboids and trapezius, which adduct the shoulder blades. The rotator cuff muscles (supraspinatus, infraspinatus, subscapularis, teres minor) act to keep the humerus in neutral alignment, while the posterior deltoids and triceps extend the shoulders and elbows. The pronators in the forearms and the intrinsic muscles of the hand distribute pressure through the whole hand to protect the heel of the hand and decrease pressure in the wrist.

Lengthening

Spine: Rectus abdominis, obliques, psoas major, sternocleidomastoid, suprahyoid, and infrahyoid.

Legs: Rectus femoris, iliacus, and psoas major.

Arms: Biceps, pectoralis major and minor, coracobrachialis, anterior deltoids, subclavius.

Rib cage: Internal intercostals, transversus thoracis, serratus posterior inferior.

Obstacles and Notes

If the goal is to have extension distributed throughout the whole spine, there will need to be more action in the thoracic region and less in the lumbar and cervical regions. This translates into concentric work for the extensors in the thoracic spine and eccentric work for the flexors in the cervical and lumbar spines.

The latissimus dorsi are not so helpful in this pose, because they can fix the scapulae on the rib cage and inhibit extension in the thoracic spine. They also produce internal rotation of the humerus and downward rotation of the scapulae, which oppose the actions of upward-facing dog.

Depending on where restrictions are, the humerus can be pulled into either internal or external rotation. Sometimes the external rotation that is active in downward-facing dog needs to be modulated coming into upward-facing dog, because the whole hand–scapula relationship shifts relative to the spine.

Breathing

As the counterpose to the "exhaled" downward-facing dog, this pose is clearly related to the expansive action of inhaling.

Many who practice Ashtanga-based sequencing experience this pose only for half a breath, as they move through it between chaturanga dandasana and downward-facing dog. Holding it for several breaths allows the inhaling action to deepen the extension in the thoracic spine, whereas the exhaling action can assist in stabilizing the lumbar and cervical curves.

Adho Mukha Vrksasana

Downward-Facing Tree Pose

ah-doh moo-kah vriks-SHAHS-anna

adho mukha = face downward

vrksa = tree

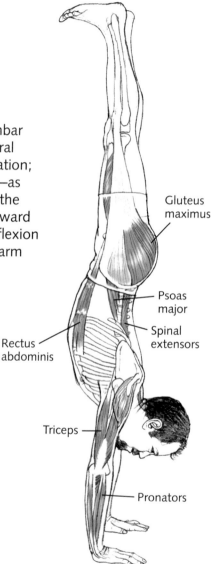

Classification and Level

Advanced inverted arm support

Joint Actions

Spine cervical extension, slight thoracic and lumbar extension; neutral sacroiliac joints; hips neutral extension, adduction, and slight internal rotation; knee extension; ankle neutral (dorsi)flexion—as opposed to the gymnastic version, in which the toes are pointed (plantarflexion); scapula upward rotation and abduction; glenohumeral joint flexion and external rotation; elbow extension; forearm pronation; wrist dorsiflexion.

Working

Legs: Gravity tries to flex and abduct the hips, so to maintain neutral extension, the hamstrings are active, along with the adductor magnus to maintain adduction, internal rotation, and extension.

The iliacus and psoas major work to resist hyperextension in the lumbar spine from the legs falling back. The abdominal muscles are quite active, particularly the transversus and obliques to stabilize the spine. The spinal extensors act to lift into the pose, and to maintain balance once there. The gluteus maximus also helps to lift the legs into the pose, but does not need to be too active to maintain it.

Arms: As in downward-facing dog, the serratus anterior creates upward rotation and stabilization of the scapulae on the rib cage. The deltoids flex the shoulder; the infraspinatus, teres minor, and posterior deltoids maintain external rotation in the glenohumeral joint. The triceps maintain extension of the elbows and the pronators rotate the forearms to balance the rotation of the humerus; flexor carpi radialis and ulnaris protect the carpal tunnel. The intrinsic muscles of the hand work to maintain the hand's arches.

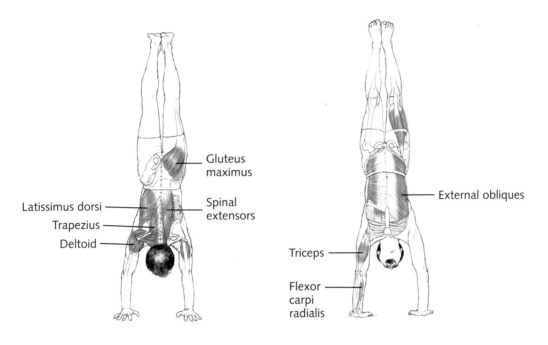

Gluteus maximus

Latissimus dorsi

Trapezius

Deltoid

Spinal extensors

External obliques

Triceps

Flexor carpi radialis

Obstacles and Notes

If the latissimus dorsi are tight, the flexion and upward rotation of the arms can cause hyperextension in the lumbar spine.

Hands and wrists alert: It's very challenging to maintain the integrity of the hands with all the weight of the body balancing on them, but it's essential in this pose, because collapsing into the wrist or heel of the hand is quite dangerous for the carpal tunnel and the nerves passing through it.

Overuse of the gluteus maximus and latissimus dorsi can create more of a banana-shaped pose, which is admittedly easier for balance and may feel more stable for many people. Doing a handstand with a neutral spine is far more challenging and recruits more core muscular strength.

For hypermobile students, it is especially important to find the strength of deep, intrinsic muscles, so that the pose doesn't become rigid, but is both stable and fluid . . . available for breathing.

Breathing

Handstand is one of the most difficult poses in which to breathe effectively. The combined action of the core supporting muscles, working to minimize shape change in the spine, also minimizes the breath movements. Add to this the challenges of balancing, inversion, and strong upper-body action, and breathing is likely to be relegated to an afterthought at best.

Many people instinctively hold their breath in handstand, partly out of fear, but also because of a need to stabilize the movements of the spine. Of course, to maintain this balance for more than a few seconds, the breath must be integrated into the pose—not necessarily as deep, full breaths, but as quick, efficient breaths that don't disrupt the balancing or stabilizing actions of the core musculature.

Chaturanga Dandasana

Four-Limbed Stick Pose

chaht-tour-ANG-ah don-DAHS-anna

chatur = four

anga = limb

danda = staff, stick

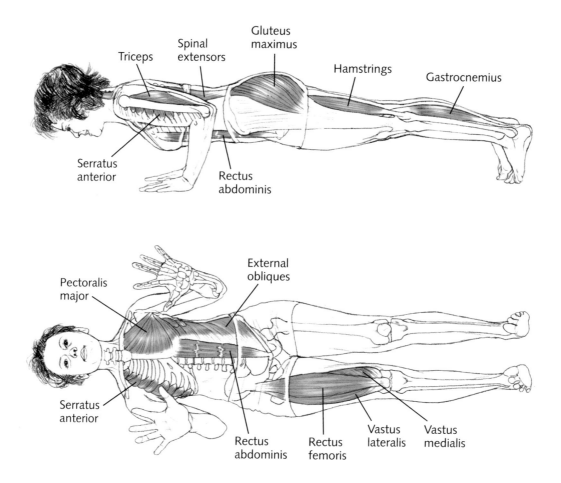

Classification and Level

Intermediate arm support in axial extension

Joint Actions

Neutral spine; neutral sacroiliac joint; hip adduction, internal rotation, neutral extension; knee flexion; ankle dorsiflexion; neutral scapula; neutral glenohumeral joint; elbow flexion; forearm pronation; wrist extension.

Working

Gravity.

Stabilizing spine: Obliques, rectus abdominis, psoas minor, eccentrically; spinal muscles, especially the cervical spine, concentrically.

Legs: Hamstrings; adductor magnus; some gluteus maximus, concentrically; psoas major; iliacus; rectus femoris, eccentrically, for neutral hip extension; vastii and articularis genus, for knee extension; gastrocnemius and soleus modulate tibialis anterior to create dorsiflexion; intrinsic and extrinsic foot muscles.

Arms: Serratus anterior, eccentrically, to prevent winging of the scapula; rotator cuff (subscapularis to protect the front of the joint, mainly infraspinatus and teres minor to externally rotate the humerus against the pull of the pectoralis and coracobrachialis); pectoralis major, pectoralis minor, coracobrachialis, and triceps, eccentrically; pronators; intrinsic and extrinsic hand muscles.

Notes

Weakness in the pose shows up in the lower body as lumbar hyperextension combined with hip flexion. To counter this, the coordinated action of the hamstrings is important.

In the upper body, weakness in the triceps and serratus anterior can show up as a downward rotation of the scapulae and an overuse of the pectoralis major and minor.

Depressing the scapulae by recruiting the latisssimus dorsi can give a feeling of strength in the back, but it contributes to hyperextension of the lumbar spine and a downward rotation of the scapulae.

Breathing

Maintaining this position relative to gravity calls into play virtually all the respiratory muscles, along with the arms and shoulder girdle. This degree of muscular effort produces a strong stabilizing effect on the movements of the diaphragm, which will operate against considerable resistance. Progress in this pose consists of making the muscular effort as efficient as possible, which will result in the ability to maintain both the alignment and smooth breathing for increasingly longer periods of time.

Astavakrasana

Eight-Angle Pose

ah-SHTA-vak-RAHS-anna

ashta = eight *vakra* = crooked, curved, bent

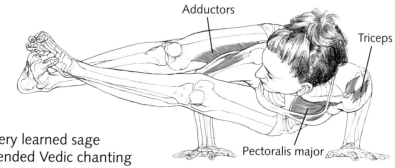

Astavakra was a very learned sage whose mother attended Vedic chanting classes while pregnant. While he was in his mother's womb, he winced at eight of his father's mispronunciations of Vedic prayers, and was thus born with eight bends in his body.

Classification and Level

Intermediate, twisting arm balance

Joint Actions

Spine cervical extension and rotation; thoracic, lumbar, and sacral flexion and rotation (head turned toward the legs, upper thorax turned away from the legs, pelvis turned toward the legs); sacroiliac joint nutation; scapula downward rotation, abduction; glenohumeral joint external rotation, adduction; elbow flexion; forearm pronation; wrist dorsiflexion; hip flexion, adduction, external rotation to enter pose and then internal rotation to seal bind; knee flexion moving toward extension; ankle dorsiflexion; foot eversion.

Working

Gravity.

Spine: Psoas minor, abdominal muscles, and pelvic floor, for flexion; top-leg external obliques, rotatores, and multifidi, for rotation; bottom-leg internal obliques and erector spinae; top-side quadratus lumborum, to keep hips from dropping to the floor; bottom-leg-side sternocleidomastoid; top-leg-side splenius capitis, to rotate the head.

Legs: Psoas major and iliacus, to flex hips; pectineus, adductor longus, and adductor brevis, to adduct and flex the hips; adductor magnus, to adduct and internally rotate the legs; rectus femoris, to flex the hips and extend the knees; vastii, to extend the knees; tibialis anterior, to dorsiflex the ankles; peroneal muscles, to dorsiflex and evert the feet.

Arms: Infraspinatus and teres minor, to externally rotate the humerus; subscapularis, supraspinatus, long head of biceps, and anterior deltoid, eccentrically, to protect the front of the shoulder joint; coracobrachialis, pectoralis major, and pectoralis minor, to abduct and downwardly rotate the scapulae; serratus anterior, to abduct the scapulae; triceps (work against gravity); flexor carpi radialis and ulnaris; intrinsic muscles of the hand.

Lengthening

Spine: Bottom-leg-side external obliques and erector spinae; top-leg-side internal obliques, rotatores, and multifidi; top-leg-side sternocleidomastoid; bottom-leg-side splenius capitis.

Legs: Hamstrings with hip flexion and knee extension; gluteus maximus, medius, and minimus with hip flexion and adduction; gastrocnemius and soleus with ankle dorsiflexion.

Arms: Rhomboids; trapezius; long head of biceps, anterior deltoid, subscapularis, and supraspinatus, eccentrically; pectoralis minor and coracobrachialis, perhaps eccentrically depending on how abducted the scapulae are.

Obstacles and Notes

This pose is a variation of parsva bakasana (addressed later in this chapter). It requires the same action in the spine, although the spine is often slightly more extended (toward neutral) in astavakrasana, which allows for a more even distribution of the rotation through the spine.

In astavakrasana, the binding of the feet keeps the legs symmetrical. This symmetry in the legs and hip joints means that the rotation has to happen more in the spine and less in the hip joints. With the wrapping of the legs around the arm, less twist is needed than in parsva bakasana, because the bottom leg doesn't have to reach quite as far. In parsva bakasana, the legs can release asymmetrically as the underneath leg slides forward, and the hip joints contribute to the rotational action of the spine.

As in ardha matsyendrasana, if the spine does not rotate, potentially risky compensatory twisting can occur through abduction or adduction of the scapulae on the rib cage.

Also, the wrapping of the legs around the arms creates a fairly stable pivot point. The challenge of this pose (if one can do parsva bakasana) is more about balance and flexibility than strength. The extended legs in this pose make the counterbalance on the support of the arms challenging.

Breathing

As compared to side crane, in which the body weight is lifted and supported on the upper arms, astavakrasana requires you to "hang" the weight of the lower body off the support of the upper arm. It's interesting to examine which pose affords easier breathing. Which pose requires more or less expenditure of energy, and which offers more freedom of movement for the diaphragm?

Bakasana

Crane Pose

bak-AHS-anna

baka = crane, heron

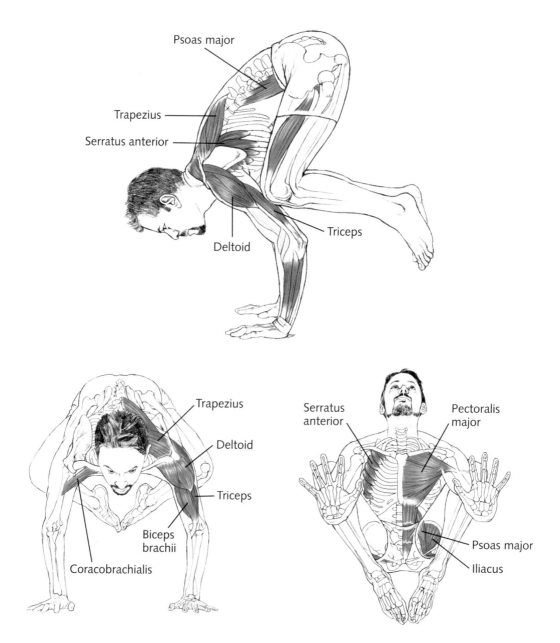

Psoas major

Trapezius

Serratus anterior

Deltoid

Triceps

Trapezius

Deltoid

Triceps

Biceps brachii

Coracobrachialis

Serratus anterior

Pectoralis major

Psoas major

Iliacus

Classification and Level

Intermediate arm balance

Joint Actions

Cervical extension of the spine; thoracic and lumbar flexion; sacrum joint nutation; hip flexion, external rotation, adduction; knee flexion; scapula downward rotation, abduction; glenohumeral joint external rotation, flexion, adduction; elbow flexion moving toward extension; forearm pronation; wrist dorsiflexion.

Working

Spine: Maintaining spinal flexion are the psoas major and minor, abdominal muscles, and pelvic floor. The deep intrinsic muscles in the posterior neck need to find cervical extension while maintaining thoracic flexion, which is a challenge because cervical extension tends to flatten the thoracic curve.

Legs: The psoas and iliacus work to flex the hip joints. The pectineus, adductor longus, and adductor brevis both adduct and flex the hip. The gracilis adducts and flexes the hip and knee, while the hamstrings maintain knee flexion.

Arms: The infraspinatus and teres minor externally rotate the humerus; the subscapularis and supraspinatus protect the front of the shoulder joints. The anterior deltoids, coracobrachialis, and pectoralis major and minor abduct and downwardly rotate the scapulae. The serratus anterior abducts the scapulae, and the triceps work against gravity to extend the elbow. The flexor carpi radialis and ulnaris, and the intrinsic muscles of the hand, maintain the hand's arches. The arms begin in flexion, but move toward extension against gravity when lifting into the pose.

Lengthening

Spinal extensors, anterior neck muscles, rhomboids, trapezius.

Obstacles and Notes

In bird poses (eagle, crow, rooster, peacock), common factors are flexion of the thoracic spine, abduction of the scapulae, and extension of the cervical spine. In other words, wings are spread and the beak is lifted.

These actions require precision and strength in the muscles of the spine to achieve cervical extension without engaging the trapezius, which will interfere with the action of the scapulae and arms.

Breathing

Because the thoracic region is maintained in flexion, breath movements in the rib cage are minimized in crane pose. The lower abdomen is also stabilized somewhat by the deep abdominal and hip flexor action, but the upper abdomen is relatively free to move.

(continued)

Bakasana Variation

Parsva Bakasana

parsh-vah bak-AHS-anna

Side Crane Pose

parsva = side

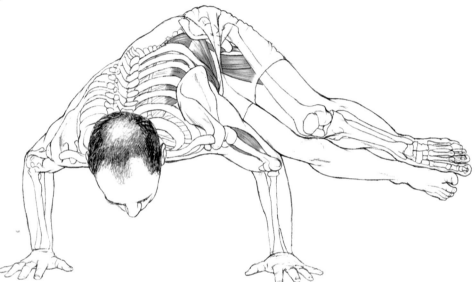

Classification and Level

Intermediate twisting arm balance

Joint Actions

Cervical extension of the spine; thoracic, lumbar, and sacral flexion and rotation; sacroiliac joint nutation; hip flexion, internal rotation, adduction; knee flexion (or extension); scapula downward rotation, abduction; glenohumeral joint external rotation, flexion, abduction; elbow flexion moving toward extension; forearm pronation; wrist dorsiflexion.

Working

Spinal flexion: Same as bakasana, but also with right internal obliques, left external obliques, right erector spinae, left rotatores, and multifidi to turn the legs to the left and axially rotate the thoracic spine.

Legs: Same as bakasana.

Arms: Same as bakasana, although the arms are abducted rather than adducted, to widen the base of the pose. It's important to maintain external rotation of the glenohumeral joint, because the work is much more asymmetrical in this pose.

Obstacles and Notes

If the knees separate in this pose, the rotation is happening more in the hip joints than in the spine.

In the rotated pose, the arms are more abducted and the spine is more extended than in bakasana.

Because this is a bound pose, it can put a lot of force into the lower back when it is in a vulnerable position. That force comes not only from the knees on the arm, but also from the weight of the body.

Breathing

Similar as in bakasana, but even more restricted because of the twisting of the spine.

Mayurasana

Peacock Pose

ma-yur-AHS-anna

mayura = peacock

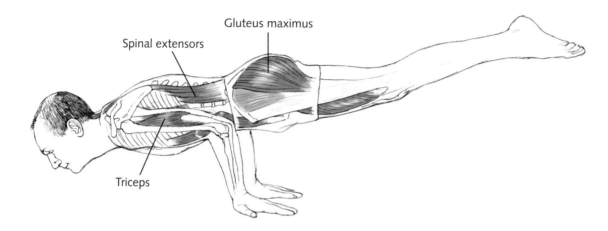

Spinal extensors

Gluteus maximus

Triceps

Classification and Level

Advanced extended arm balance

Joint Actions

Cervical extension of the spine; mild thoracic flexion; mild lumbar extension; hip extension, adduction, internal rotation; knee extension; ankle plantarflexion; scapula downward rotation and abduction; glenohumeral joint external rotation, flexion, adduction; elbow flexion; forearm supination; wrist dorsiflexion.

Working

Spine: Psoas major and minor and abdominal muscles resist the pressure of the elbows into the viscera; pelvic floor muscles; deep intrinsic muscles in the neck to find cervical extension while maintaining thoracic flexion; all spinal extensors (especially in the lumbar region, to help lift the legs).

Legs: Hamstrings, to extend the hips; adductor magnus, to extend, internally rotate, and adduct; gluteus medius, minimus, and maximus, to help with extension.

Arms: Infraspinatus and teres minor, to externally rotate the humerus; subscapularis and supraspinatus, to protect the front of the joint; anterior deltoids, coracobrachialis, pectoralis major, and pectoralis minor, to abduct and downwardly rotate the scapulae; serratus anterior, to abduct the scapulae; triceps, against gravity, to extend the elbow; extensor carpi radialis and ulnaris; intrinsic muscles of the hand.

Lengthening

Anterior neck muscles, rhomboids, trapezius.

Obstacles and Notes

As in the other bird poses (eagle, crow, rooster), peacock involves flexion of the thoracic spine, abduction of the scapulae, and extension of the cervical spine. It's unusual to balance on the arms with the forearms supinated. This changes the action in the wrist, because the extensors are more active to resist plantarflexion (falling into gravity).

Breathing

The pressure of the elbows into the abdomen stimulates the organs. Many benefits have traditionally been ascribed to this effect. All the abdominal muscles produce a strong isometric contraction to resist the pressure of the elbows into the viscera. Although no hip flexion is involved in peacock, the psoas muscle also works strongly from behind the peritoneum, to reduce the pressure on the anterior lumbar spine. So, the abdominal organs are being strongly squeezed from front and back—as well as from above and below—by the respiratory and pelvic diaphragms.

Considering how much muscular energy is expended to maintain this pose, and the minimal amount of breathing it permits, it's no wonder that it is rarely held for more than a few moments. The lungs in their limited capacity are simply unable to supply enough oxygen for that degree of muscular effort.

A variation of mayurasana with legs in padmasana (lotus), is actually easier to maintain. This is due to the reduced muscular effort of stabilizing the lower body and the necessary repositioning of the elbows into the upper abdomen. This position takes less energy to stabilize than when the elbows press into the lower abdomen (which is the balance point when the legs are fully extended).

Pincha Mayurasana

Feathered Peacock Pose

pin-cha ma-yur-AHS-anna

pincha = a feather of a tail

mayura = peacock

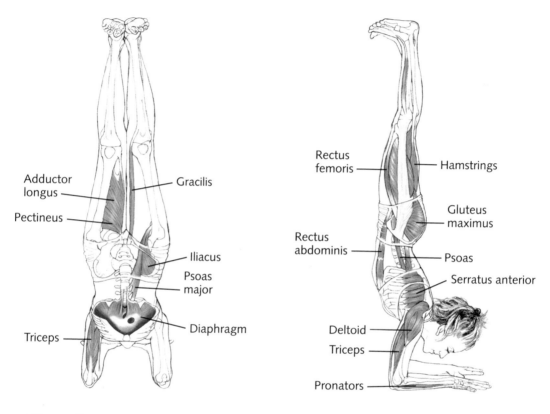

Adductor longus

Gracilis

Pectineus

Iliacus

Psoas major

Triceps

Diaphragm

Rectus femoris

Hamstrings

Gluteus maximus

Rectus abdominis

Psoas

Serratus anterior

Deltoid

Triceps

Pronators

Classification and Level

Advanced inverted arm support

Joint Actions

Extension is maintained throughout spine: The more extension there is in the thoracic spine, the less there will have to be in the cervical and lumbar spines. Neutral hip extension; knee extension; ankle neutral dorsiflexion; scapula abduction, upward rotation, and elevation; glenohumeral joint flexion, external rotation, and adduction; elbow flexion; and forearm pronation.

Working

Spine: Intrinsic muscles of the spine (intertransversarii, interspinalis, rotatores, multifidi); most spinal extensors (spinalis, semispinalis, longissimus dorsi, iliocostalis). Psoas minor, obliques, rectus abdominis, and transversus abdominis are very active eccentrically in the pose, to keep from falling backward.

Legs: Adductor magnus and hamstrings, to hold the legs together and extend the hips; vastii, to extend the knees.

Arms: Serratus anterior, to abduct and upwardly rotate the scapulae; infraspinatus and teres minor, to externally rotate the arms; subscapularis and supraspinatus with infraspinatus and teres minor, to stabilize the humerus in the glenoid fossa; anterior deltoids, pectoralis major and coracobrachialis, to adduct and flex the arm; triceps, eccentrically, to resist the flexion of the elbows (and crashing into the face); pronators of the forearms, to bring the wrists flat on the floor.

Lengthening

Latissimus dorsi, iliacus, rectus femoris, forearm supinators, abdominal muscles, internal intercostals (due to rib cage expansion and thoracic extension), anterior neck muscles.

Obstacles and Notes

If the rotator cuff is active, the glenohumeral joint is stabilized, and the scapulae are more free to mobilize on the rib cage (with the serratus anterior), there will also be more freedom in the thoracic spine to extend and in the rib cage to breathe. Mobility in the thoracic spine is important; much like in upward-facing dog, the more extension there is in the thoracic spine, the less the lower back and cervical spine have to do.

The triceps and deltoids are eccentrically very active, to resist falling forward onto the face or head. This is a great preparation pose for handstand, because it strengthens the arms.

If tightness in the forearm (either in the supinators or in the interosseus membrane between the radius and the ulna) restricts full pronation, the elbows will swing open or the hands will come together. This common forearm issue is often interpreted as tightness in the shoulders or weakness in the wrists.

Shortness in the latissimus dorsi can also pull the elbows wide, by internally rotating the humerus. This can feel like tight shoulders, but can actually be addressed by side bending and other actions that lengthen the latissimus dorsi. Shortness in these muscles will also cause too much lumbar extension and interfere with breathing.

Breathing

The base of support for this pose is formed by the forearms, rib cage, and thoracic spine, and these structures need to be quite stable to maintain balance. Because of this, excessive chest breathing interferes with supporting a forearm stand. On the other hand, the weight of the legs and pelvis and the curve of the lumbar spine need to be stabilized by the abdominal muscles, making too much abdominal movement counterproductive. Because of these factors, a breathing pattern that moves equally and smoothly throughout the body is needed.

Purvottanasana

Upward Plank Pose

POOR-vo-tan-AHS-ahna

purva = front, east

ut = intense

tan = extend, stretch

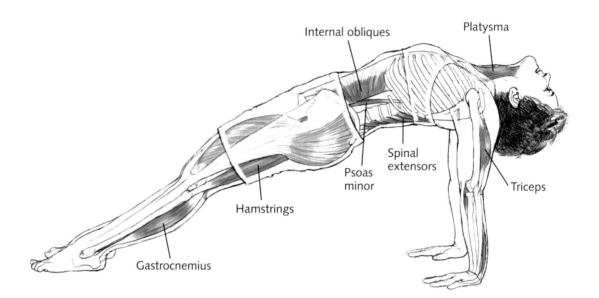

Internal obliques · Platysma · Spinal extensors · Psoas minor · Triceps · Hamstrings · Gastrocnemius

Classification and Level

Basic backbending arm support

Joint Actions

Spinal extension; sacroiliac counternutation; hip extension, internal rotation, and adduction; knee extension; ankle plantarflexion; toe extension; scapula adduction, downward rotation, elevation; glenohumeral joint extension, neutral rotation (some people need to internally rotate and some people need to externally rotate their humerus to maintain neutral alignment); elbow extension; forearm pronation; wrist extension; finger extension.

Working

Spine: Throughout the spine the extensors are active, although they are most active in the thoracic spine. Gravity does much of the work of extension in the lumbar spine, so the psoas minor can be active eccentrically to resist too much lumbar lordosis. The obliques do the same.

In the cervical spine, gravity creates the extension, and the anterior neck muscles (longus capitis, longus colli, and so forth) can work eccentrically to keep the forces in the neck balanced. In the thoracic spine, semispinalis thoracis, spinalis thoracis, the thoracic part of interspinalis, and the rotatores are the most active.

Legs: To extend the hips, the hamstrings should be primary, perhaps assisted by the extensor portion of the gluteus maximus. The adductor magnus creates internal rotation, extension, and adduction; the gracilis can help with adduction. The vastii and articularis genus work to extend the knees; the gastrocnemius and soleus plantarflex the ankle, while the intrinsic and extrinsic foot muscles extend the toes.

Arms: The teres major, posterior deltoids, and triceps work to extend the humerus, with the rhomboids and trapezius acting to maintain adduction. The rotator cuff muscles (supraspinatus, infraspinatus, subscapularis, teres minor) act to keep the humerus in neutral alignment. The triceps extend the elbows, while the pronators of the forearm and the intrinsic muscles of the hand distribute weight through the whole hand. This protects the heel of the hand from too much pressure.

Lengthening

Spine: Rectus abdominis, obliques, psoas major, sternocleidomastoid, suprahyoid and infrahyoid muscles; psoas minor and obliques.

Legs: Rectus femoris, iliacus, and psoas major.

Arms: Serratus anterior, biceps, pectoralis major and minor, coracobrachialis, anterior deltoid subclavius.

Obstacles and Notes

Often in this pose there is too much lumbar extension and not enough hip extension. The hamstrings should be the main extensors here, but if they are weak, the gluteus maximus can kick in. A problem with this, however, is that it brings in external rotation, which is harder on the lower back. The gluteus maximus can also overdo the lumbar extension.

If the hamstrings are too weak to do purvottanasana, then tabletop (chatus pada pitham, discussed later in this chapter) is a great preparation.

The latissimus dorsi are not so helpful in this pose, because they can fix the scapulae on the rib cage and inhibit extension in the thoracic spine.

Breathing

It's an interesting challenge to downwardly rotate the scapulae and still extend the spine. This is because depressing the scapulae tends to create flexion in the spine. The solution to this dilemma is to allow the breathing movements to mobilize the upper rib cage and sternum, which will deepen the extension in the upper back from the front line of the body.

Salamba Sirsasana

Supported Headstand

sah-LOM-bah shear-SHAHS-anna

sa = with

alamba = that on which one rests or leans, support

sirsa = head

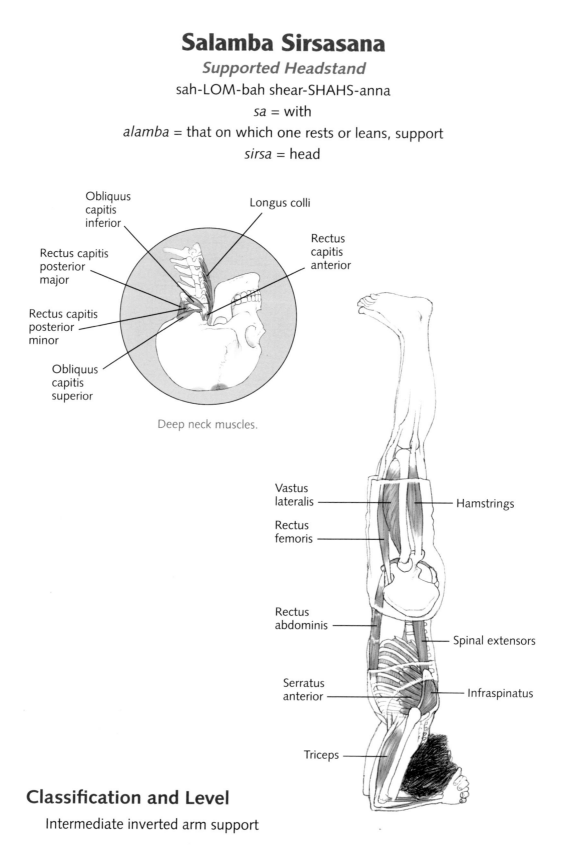

Obliquus capitis inferior

Longus colli

Rectus capitis anterior

Rectus capitis posterior major

Rectus capitis posterior minor

Obliquus capitis superior

Deep neck muscles.

Vastus lateralis

Hamstrings

Rectus femoris

Rectus abdominis

Spinal extensors

Serratus anterior

Infraspinatus

Triceps

Classification and Level

Intermediate inverted arm support

Joint Actions

Spine neutral axial extension, or slight extension; hip extension; knee extension; ankle neutral dorsiflexion; scapula abduction, upward rotation, and elevation; glenohumeral joint flexion, external rotation, and adduction; elbow flexion; forearm in neutral rotation.

Weight Placement

For some, the ideal placement of the weight on the skull is on the bregma—the juncture between the coronal and sagittal sutures, where the frontal bone meets the two parietal bones. This leads to a slightly more arched final position.

Placing the weight more toward the crown of the head leads to a more neutral spine and more balanced action between the front and back of the body.

Working

Spine: The intrinsic muscles of the spine (intertransversarii, interspinalis, rotatores, multifidi, spinalis, semispinalis, splenius capitis and cervicis, longissimus, and iliocostalis) are all active to lift up into headstand, and to prevent falling down forward. Entering the pose demands work in the extensors of the thoracic spine, which may be unaccustomed to lifting the weight of the whole lower body. The psoas minor, obliques, rectus abdominis, and transversus are very active in the pose, to keep from falling backward. The pelvic diaphragm also is drawn into action along with the lower abdominal muscles, creating a strong mula bandha effect.

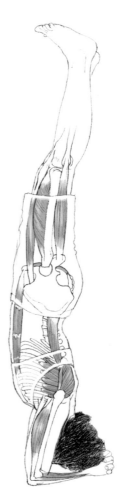

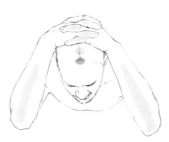

Supporting the weight on the bregma—the darker blue spot in left illustration—results in a slightly more arched position (right). Supporting weight near the crown—lighter blue spot—leads to a more neutral spine position.

(continued)

Salamba Sirsasana   *(continued)*

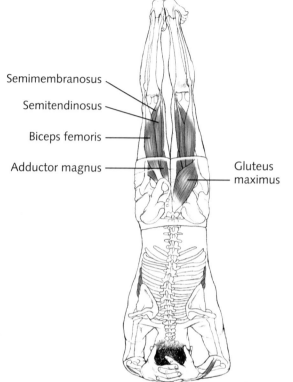

Semimembranosus

Semitendinosus

Biceps femoris

Adductor magnus

Gluteus maximus

The author's scoliosis is exaggerated in sirsasana.

Neck: The rectus capitis anterior, rectus capitis posterior major and minor, obliquus capitis superior and inferior, longus capitis, and longus colli all work to balance the front and back of the atlanto-occipital joint and the atlanto-axial joint.

Arms: Serratus anterior acts to wrap the scapulae; infraspinatus and teres minor externally rotate the arms; and supraspinatus and subscapularis help hold the head of the humerus in its socket. The triceps are active to stabilize the elbows as the extensor and flexor carpi ulnaris press the little finger side of the hands into the floor.

Legs: The adductor magnus and hamstrings act to hold the legs together and extend the hip joints. The vastii extend the knees, and the medial fibers of gluteus maximus extend the hips (without external rotation).

Obstacles and Notes

Spine: Many people have asymmetries and slight rotations in their spines, which become more apparent in this pose. Note the rotational shifts, scoliosis, and other asymmetries in the illustration of the author in sirsasana.

Neck: If the deep muscles of the neck are accessed, the jaw and vocal muscles are able to stay relaxed.

Legs: It can be a challenge to find full hip extension in this pose. If the abdominal muscles are not strong enough, the hips can flex to keep the work of the pose in the back muscles instead of in the front.

Note: Contrary to popular notions of increased blood or oxygen flow to the brain in inversions, it should be noted that the body has very robust mechanisms that control the amount of blood delivered to any given region—irrespective of the orientation to gravity.

Regional changes in *blood pressure* have been observed based on inversion or compression of major blood vessels by body position, but this is a distinct issue from movement of blood volume and thus oxygen delivery.

That said, inversions do offer a very beneficial opportunity for increased venous return from the lower body, as well as improved lymph drainage—not to mention the benefits derived from inverting the action of the diaphragm.

Technique

Even if you favor the "bregma" version of this pose, and enter into the pose with straight legs with the intention to end up in a more arched position, the strength and coordination required to maintain headstand safely demands certain skills that can be best developed by practicing the bent-leg entry into the pose. The key test is whether you can raise the weight off the feet without jumping, and maintain the difficult pose known as acunchanasana for several breaths.

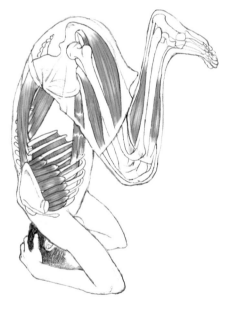

Acunchanasana.

Breathing

When the support for sirsasana is derived from the deeper intrinsic muscles of the spine, as well as the coordinated action of the hamstrings, vastii, psoas minor, internal obliques, transversus abdominis, and serratus anterior, the weight forces of the body will be more neutralized in gravity. Then, the muscular effort of remaining in the pose will be minimized, and the breath will be calm and efficient. At that point, the inverted nature of the diaphragm's action is emphasized because of the strong action of the abdominal muscles and pelvic diaphragm, which help to stabilize the center of gravity over the base of support. All the internal organs, which anchor to the central tendon of the diaphragm, can move differently in inversions.

Vrschikasana

Scorpion Pose

vrs-chee-KAHS-anna

vrschana = scorpion

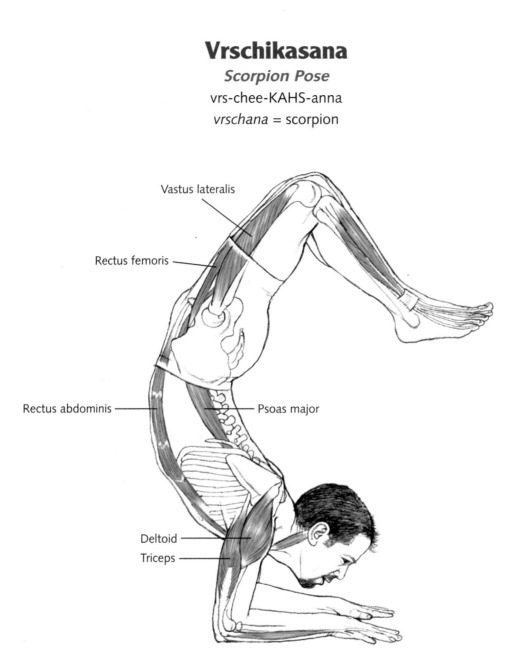

Vastus lateralis

Rectus femoris

Rectus abdominis

Psoas major

Deltoid

Triceps

Classification and Level

Intermediate inverted arm balance

Joint Actions

Full spinal extension; hip extension, adduction, internal rotation; knee flexion; ankle neutral dorsiflexion; scapula adduction, upward rotation; glenohumeral joint external rotation, flexion, adduction; elbow flexion; forearm pronation.

Working

Same as pincha mayurasana. In addition, the hamstrings flex the knees and draw the toes down to the head (if the person is flexible enough in the front line of body—otherwise, the legs hang passively in position). The serratus anterior works eccentrically as the scapulae adduct. Spinal extensors work to deepen extension and lift the head against gravity and toward the feet.

Lengthening

Similar to pincha mayurasana. Latissimus dorsi, iliacus, rectus femoris, forearm supinators, abdominal muscles, internal intercostals, anterior neck muscles. The rectus femoris and muscles of the anterior torso especially stretch; vastii lengthen with knee flexion, and pectoralis major and minor may lengthen with thoracic extension and scapula adduction.

Obstacles and Notes

Even though pincha mayurasana is considered preparation for vrschikasana, scorpion is actually an easier pose to maintain because of its lower center of gravity.

To deepen from pincha mayurasana into scorpion, the scapulae need to slide together on the back, which lowers the rib cage toward the floor and creates more mobility in the thoracic spine. The head then can lift and the thoracic spine can extend further. This also changes the balance point from between the shoulders to further caudal in the spine, made necessary by the bending of the knees.

The lifting of the head is important to shifting the balance point; otherwise, the legs might overbalance the pose backward, causing you to fall into a backbend.

As the knees bend actively toward the head, the hamstrings are in the shortest working length. For this reason, they often cramp while trying to do this action.

As important as getting into this pose is the ability to get out of it and find the relative neutrality of pincha mayurasana again. It's a good idea to practice it in a manageable range—entering and exiting the pose with control. This is a good challenge because it gets muscles at maximum length to contract concentrically.

Breathing

Breathing in this pose is similar to breathing in pincha mayurasana, except that the abdominal breath movement is limited by the stretch of the muscles there, rather than by their stabilizing contraction.

Urdhva Dhanurasana

Upward Bow Pose, Wheel Pose

OORD-vah don-your-AHS-anna

urdhva = upward

dhanu = bow

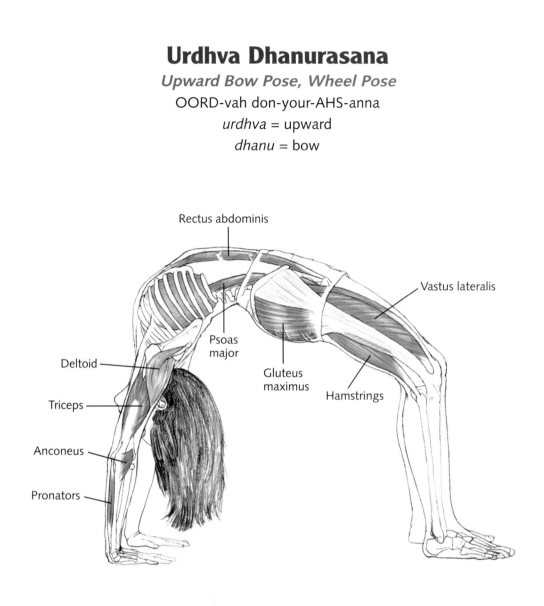

Rectus abdominis

Vastus lateralis

Psoas major

Deltoid

Gluteus maximus

Triceps

Hamstrings

Anconeus

Pronators

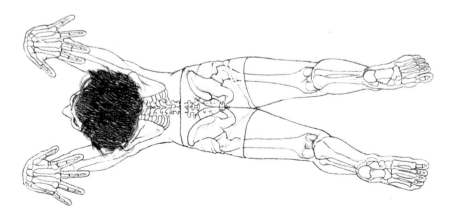

Classification and Level

Intermediate inverted backbend

Joint Actions

Full-spine extension; sacroiliac counternutation; hip extension, internal rotation, adduction; knee extension; ankle dorsiflexion; scapula upward rotation, abduction (deepens into scapular adduction with more thoracic extension); glenohumeral flexion, external rotation, adduction; elbow extension; forearm pronation; wrist dorsiflexion.

Working

Spine: All the spinal extensors through the length of the spine are active, especially the deeper layers: interspinalis, intertransversarii, rotatores, multifidi, transversospinalis group. The psoas minor and abdominal muscles work eccentrically to resist overmobilizing the lumbar spine, and encourage extension in the thoracic spine.

Legs: The hamstrings work to extend the hips; the adductor magnus extends, internally rotates, and adducts the hips (the other adductors are less helpful because they tend to pull the hips into flexion). The gluteus maximus helps to extend the hips, but too much gluteus action will also externally rotate the legs; vastii extend the knees.

Arms: The infraspinatus, teres minor, and posterior deltoids create external rotation at the glenohumeral joint, and the subscapularis protects the front of the joint. The serratus anterior abducts the scapulae and elevates the arms; the deltoids flex the arms at the shoulders, and the triceps and anconeus extend the elbows. The coracobrachialis flexes and adducts the arms at the shoulders. The pronators in the forearms turn the palms toward the floor.

Lengthening

Legs: Rectus femoris, psoas major, and iliacus.

Torso: Abdominal muscles and anterior rib cage muscles, primarily internal intercostals and anterior neck muscles.

Arms: Pectoralis major and minor, latissimus dorsi.

(continued)

Urdhva Dhanurasana   *(continued)*

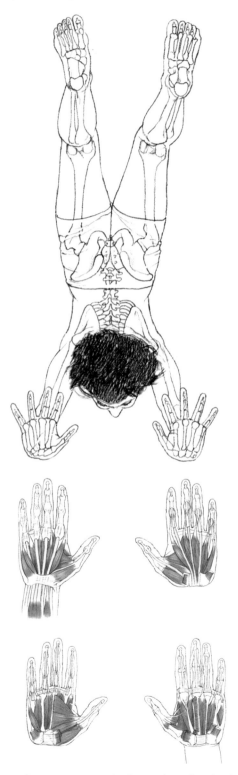

Hand musculature mirroring the layers found in the foot (page 37).

Obstacles and Notes

Overall, the correct leg action is critical to getting into the upward bow. Most people instinctively use their quadriceps in a pushing action, which thrusts weight toward the head and arms, making it very difficult to raise the upper body off the floor. Initiating the lift of the pelvis with more of a "pulling" action resolves this difficulty.

One of the challenges to accomplishing this is to use the hip extensors to support the action in the legs, rather than the quadriceps as knee extensors. The strength of the hamstrings and adductor magnus can significantly decrease the work in the quadriceps.

Of the adductor group, the adductor magnus is most useful for upward bow, because it creates hip extension and internal rotation along with adduction—all actions that support the alignment of the pose. The gluteus maximus is less useful for hip extension in this position, because it can create external rotation, which can lead to compression in the sacrum and lower-back pain.

The arms need to move freely overhead, and a combination of mobilizing the scapulae and stabilizing the external rotation in the shoulder joints with the rotator cuff creates the necessary balance. If the latissimus dorsi are tight, they will restrict the ability of the scapulae to upwardly rotate. This can force excessive action into the spine or shoulder joints.

Similarly, if there is restriction in hip extension, too much of the action can accumulate in the lumbar spine.

Breathing

Many students have been frustrated by their inability to take deep, full breaths in urdhva dhanurasana. The reason for this is simple: In this shape, the body is stabilized in a maximal inhalation, and there is very little one can do to expand further if attempting to inhale deeply. Quiet, relaxed breathing is preferable. The more efficient the muscle action in the pose is, the less oxygen you'll need to fuel the effort.

Vasisthasana

Side Plank Pose (Sage Vasistha's Pose)

vah-sish-TAHS-anna

vasistha = a sage; most excellent, best, richest

Classification and Level

Basic one-arm balance

Joint Actions

Spine neutral; hip neutral extension, adduction, and internal rotation; knee extension; ankle dorsiflexion and feet everted against the pull of gravity; scapula neutral (abducting against the pull of gravity); glenohumeral lateral abduction, external rotation; elbow extension; bottom hand—forearm pronation, wrist dorsiflexion; top hand—forearm neutral, wrist neutral extension.

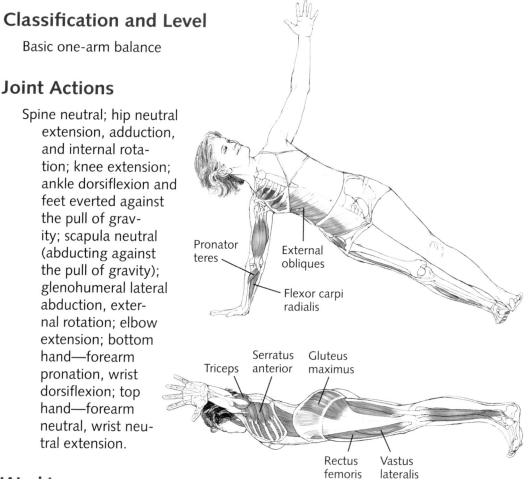

Pronator teres

External obliques

Flexor carpi radialis

Triceps

Serratus anterior

Gluteus maximus

Rectus femoris

Vastus lateralis

Working

Spine: Spinal extensors, abdominal obliques, rectus abdominis, and transversus, to maintain the neutral curves of the spine; quadratus lumborum, to resist the hips dropping to the floor; bottom-side sternocleidomastoid and top-side splenius capitis, to turn the head upward.

Torso: Top side: external obliques, concentrically, to resist the hips twisting forward; internal obliques, eccentrically, to resist the hips falling back. Bottom side: internal obliques, concentrically, to draw the right hip forward; external obliques, eccentrically, to resist the hips falling back.

Legs: Top leg: adductor magnus, to internally rotate and extend the hips; hamstrings, to extend the hips; vastii, to extend the knees; tibialis anterior, to dorsiflex the ankles; extensor digitorum, to extend the toes. Bottom leg: adductor magnus, to internally rotate and extend the hips; hamstrings, to extend the hips; gluteus medius and minimus, to hold the hips off the floor; vastii, to extend the knees; tibialis anterior and extensor digitorum, to dorsiflex the ankles and extend the toes; peroneal muscles, to evert the foot against gravity.

Arms: Top arm: infraspinatus and teres minor, to externally rotate the humerus; serratus anterior, trapezius, and deltoid, to lift the arm; triceps, to extend the elbow; extensor carpi, to extend the wrist; and extensor digitorum, to extend the fingers. Bottom arm: serratus anterior, to maintain neutral scapulae against the adduction force of gravity; infraspinatus and teres minor, to externally rotate the humerus; subscapularis and supraspinatus, to stabilize the head of the humerus in the glenoid fossa; deltoid, to help stabilize the head of the humerus in the glenoid fossa; triceps, to extend the elbow; pronators in the forearm; flexor carpi ulnaris and radialis; intrinsic muscles of the hand to support the wrist and palm of the hand.

Lengthening

Latissimus dorsi, pectoralis major and minor, coracobrachialis.

Obstacles and Notes

The challenge of this pose is not one of flexibility, but instead of how to maintain the neutral alignment of the spine and legs and the simple position of the arms against the action of gravity. The asymmetrical relationship to gravity means that muscles have to work asymmetrically to create a symmetrical alignment of the body—essentially tadasana turned on its side.

There are many ways that gravity pulls the body out of tadasana in this pose: The spine may twist, the hips may fall forward or the shoulders may fall back (or vice versa), the bottom scapula and bottom leg may both adduct, and the pelvis may fall to the floor. It's easy to overcompensate by lifting the hips too high, or to create lateral flexion of the spine in either direction, by either giving in to gravity or overresisting it.

Overall, the side plank pose is very simple, but not very easy.

Breathing

From the standpoint of the breath, this pose has much in common with niralamba sarvangasana (unsupported shoulder stand). It is also a challenging balance pose that requires a lot of stabilizing action in the abdominal and thoracic musculature. Side plank is a bit easier, because the arms can be used for support and balance, but deep breathing will still have the effect of destabilizing the pose.

Efficiency—finding the minimum amount of effort necessary to maintain the position—allows the limited breath movements to supply just enough energy to sustain the pose.

Chatus Pada Pitham

Four-Footed Tabletop Pose

CHA-toos pada PEE-tham

chatur = four

pada = foot

pitham = stool, seat, chair, bench

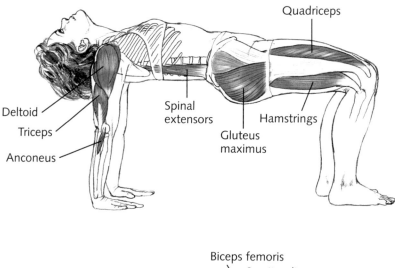

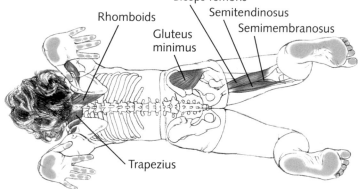

Classification and Level

Basic backbending arm support

Joint Actions

Slight lumbar and thoracic extension; cervical extension; hip neutral extension, adduction, internal rotation; knee flexion; ankle dorsiflexion; scapula downward rotation, adduction, elevation; glenohumeral joint extension and external rotation; elbow extension; forearm pronation; wrist dorsiflexion.

Working

Legs: The body weight in gravity wants to flex and abduct the hips, so the hamstrings and adductor magnus must maintain hip extension, adduction, and internal rotation. The gluteus maximus helps with hip extension but not so much that it will externally rotate the leg. The quadriceps are working eccentrically, and the tibialis anterior is drawing the knees forward, over the feet.

Arms: This is one of the few yoga poses that concentrically works the rhomboids, which along with the middle trapezius, adduct the scapulae. The levator scapulae work to elevate the scapulae. The teres major, triceps, posterior deltoids, and latissimus dorsi work to extend the arms and downwardly rotate the scapulae. The triceps extend the elbows; pronators in the forearms turn the hands toward the floor.

Torso: The abdominal muscles (obliques and rectus abdominis) and the psoas minor work to resist lumbar hyperextension from gravity.

Lengthening

Legs: Quadriceps (eccentrically), iliacus, psoas major and minor.

Torso: Abdominal muscles (all layers are working at length), anterior neck muscles.

Arms: Pectoralis major and minor, coracobrachialis.

Obstacles and Notes

Weakness in the hamstrings makes it hard to create neutral extension of the hip joints, so many people use the quadriceps to extend the knee and push the foot into the floor. The problem here is that this tends to also create hip flexion, which obstructs the opening at the front of the hip joint. Overusing the gluteus maximus will also externally rotate the hip, which the adductors will counter, creating even more restriction at the hip joint.

Too much tightness in the pectoral region will prevent the scapulae from moving into position (adduction) and will result in either too much movement in the glenohumeral joint or flexion of the spine, which will challenge the breathing.

If the chest is able to rise effectively in relation to the shoulder girdle, the base of the skull can (in most people) find a resting place on a "shelf" that's formed by the upper trapezius muscles. This can provide a very nice release of the anterior neck structures without the risk of hyperextending the cervical spine (see a similar effect in ustrasana in chapter 6).

Breathing

Unlike urdhva dhanurasana (upward bow), tabletop pose is not an extreme backbend that restricts major respiratory movements. The combination of lifting action in the back body and release in the front body makes for an interesting opportunity to experiment by moving the breath around the abdominal and thoracic regions. Some breathing patterns will have more of an effect on the stability of the pose, whereas others will assist in opening the upper rib cage.

REFERENCES AND RESOURCES

References

These are the references used for working on the poses:

Adler, S.S., D. Beckers, and M. Buck. 2003. *PNF in Practice*. 2nd ed. New York: Springer.

Clemente, C.D. 1997. *Anatomy: A Regional Atlas of the Human Body*. 4th ed. Philadelphia, PA: Lippincott Williams & Wilkins.

Gorman, David. 1995. *The Body Moveable*. 4th ed. Guelph, Ontario: Ampersand Press, 1995.

Kapit, W., and L.M. Elson. 1993. *The Anatomy Coloring Book*. 2nd ed. New York: HarperCollins College Publishers.

Kendall, F.P., E.K. McCreary, and P.G. Provance. 1993. *Muscles, Testing and Function*. 4th ed. Philadelphia, PA: Lippincott Williams & Wilkins.

Laban, R. 1966. *The Language of Movement: A Guidebook to Choreutics*. Great Britain: Macdonald and Evans.

Myers, Tom. 2001. *Anatomy Trains: Myofascial Meridians for Manual and Movement Therapists*. Churchill Livingstone.

Netter, F.H. 1997. *Atlas of Human Anatomy*. 2nd ed. East Hanover, NJ: Novartis.

Platzer, W. 2004. *Color Atlas and Textbook of Human Anatomy. Volume 1: Locomotor System*. 5th ed. New York: Thieme.

For conventional spellings of Sanskrit pronunciation, *Yoga Journal's* online resource "Pose Finder" served as an excellent guide.

For scholarly translations of Sanskrit terms, *The Cologne Digital Sanskrit Lexicon*.

Resources

Leslie Kaminoff's Yoga Anatomy Web Site—The author's personal and professional Web site containing biographical and contact information, international teaching schedule, booking information, and links to his e-Sutra blog and other writing projects: www.yogaanatomy.org

The Breathing Project, Inc.—Non-profit educational resource for breath-centered, individualized yoga founded by Leslie Kaminoff, New York, NY: www.breathingproject.org

Krishnamacharya Yoga Mandiram—The yoga of T. Krishnamacharya and his teachings, founded by T.K.V. Desikachar, Chennai, India: www.kym.org

Embodied Asana with Amy Matthews, New York, NY: www.embodiedasana.com

Gil Hedley's Somanautics Human Dissection Intensives and DVD series—Workshops taught internationally: www.somanautics.com

Tom Myers' Anatomy Trains and Kinesis Myofascial Integration—Workshops and trainings taught internationally: www.anatomytrains.com

Bonnie Bainbridge Cohen's School for Body-Mind Centering®—Developmentally-based movement reeducation and hands-on repatterning, Amherst, MA: www.bodymindcentering.com

Ron Pisaturo—Actor, writer, and a philosopher in the tradition of Aristotle and Ayn Rand: www.ronpisaturo.com

ASANA INDEXES
IN SANSKRIT AND ENGLISH

SANSKRIT INDEX

Kneeling Asanas

Supine Asanas

Prone Asanas

Arm Support Asanas

ENGLISH INDEX

Sitting Asanas

Kneeling Asanas

Supine Asanas

Prone Asanas

Arm Support Asanas

ABOUT THE AUTHOR

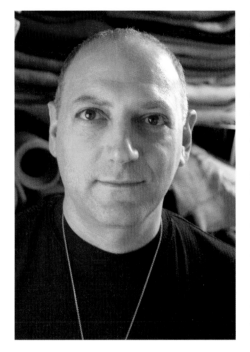

Leslie Kaminoff has more than 20 years of experience and is an internationally recognized specialist in the fields of yoga and breath anatomy. He is cofounder and head instructor of The Breathing Project, a New York City-based yoga studio dedicated to the teaching of individualized, breath-centered yoga practice and therapy.

He currently practices yoga therapy and teaches anatomy in New York City and Great Barrington, Massachusetts and advises various yoga schools on the anatomy content of their national certification program. He has led workshops for many of the leading yoga associations, schools, and training programs in the United States, and he has helped organize international yoga conferences and symposia.

Kaminoff is the founder of the highly respected international yoga list e-Sutra, and he has been a featured yoga expert in *Yoga Journal* and the *New York Times*, as well as online at WebMD, FOXNews Online, and Health.com. Kaminoff resides in Great Barrington, Massachusetts, with his wife, Uma, and their three sons.

ABOUT THE COLLABORATOR

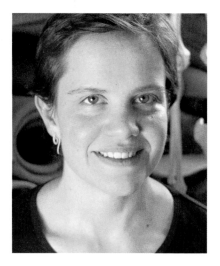

Amy Matthews, CMA, SME, RYT, RSMT/RSME, has been teaching movement since 1994. She is a Certified Laban Movement Analyst and a Body-Mind Centering™ Practitioner. Amy has been on the faculty of the Year-Long Certificate Program at the Laban/Bartenieff Institute of Movement Studies since 2000, and she teaches Embodied Asana classes and workshops at Movements Afoot, The Breathing Project, and the Society for Martial Arts Instruction in New York City.

Amy works privately as a movement therapist, integrating Laban Movement Analysis, Bartenieff Fundamentals, yoga, and Body-Mind Centering™. She coteaches "Still Moving" karate and yoga workshops with Sensei Michelle Gay for the Society for Martial Arts Instruction, and anatomy workshops for LIMS. Amy's "Embodied Asana" workshops and anatomy classes are a part of The Breathing Project's Advanced Studies Program, and she coteaches with Alison West on Yoga Union's Teacher Training program.

Amy is certified as a yoga teacher by Heart of Yoga and Yoga Union, and as a Motherhand Shiatsu practitioner. She is registered with ISMETA as a Somatic Movement Therapist and Educator, and is registered at the 500-hour level through Yoga Alliance. She studies kinesthetic anatomy with Irene Dowd and BMC™ with Bonnie Bainbridge Cohen. Amy also studies yoga with Kevin Gardiner, Mark Whitwell, and Alison West, and karate with Sensei Michelle Gay.

ABOUT THE ILLUSTRATOR

Sharon Ellis has worked as a medical illustrator in New York for more than 25 years. Her award-winning illustrations have been exhibited at the New York Academy of Medicine, the Society of Illustrators, the Association of Medical Illustrators, the Rx Club, and the Spring Street Gallery in Soho. Ellis is a member of the Association of Medical Illustrators and has received the organization's Best Illustrated Surgical Book award. She was also awarded a grant from the New York Foundation of the Arts, and her work has appeared in many medical books and magazines. Ellis holds a master's degree in medical art from the University of Texas Southwestern Medical School and a master of fine art from the State University of New York. She resides in New York City.

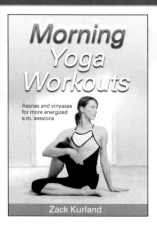
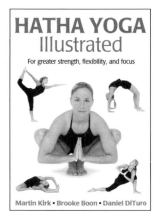
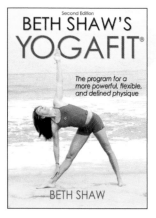